BROKEN VESSEL
RESTORED

How to Overcome Depression, Illness, Infertility, and Hormonal Imbalance and Reclaim Your Connection to God

WANDA J. COOPER

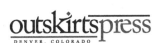

outskirtspress

DENVER, COLORADO

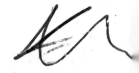

The book is dedicated to Dave—
The most loving, patient, and intelligent man I have ever known.

CONTENTS

INTRODUCTION

If you are struggling with depression, infertility, difficult pregnancies, illness, fatigue, insomnia, hormone imbalances, memory problems, or the feeling that God has abandoned you—you are not alone. For years I struggled with all these things and more. I know that there are countless women who suffer in silence. Many times the physical and emotional pains we have to endure may seem beyond our ability to bear. In my case, at these times I felt completely isolated and wondered if anyone else might be in the same situation. I vowed that if I ever found my way out of that deep, dark hole, I would share what I learned so that others wouldn't have to blindly stumble to find their own way back to health or feel so desperately alone.

If you have suffered from multiple, random symptoms of illness for any length of time it is likely that at least one doctor has made you feel like your problems were all in your head. For the record, you are not a hypochondriac. Your pains and illnesses are real, your hormone swings are real, and your mental struggles are very, very real. There is a cause for them, and even more importantly, there are solutions. As you go through the chapters of this book, you will begin to see what causes women's bodies to become sick and imbalanced and how we can heal ourselves. The solutions presented herein will empower you to take back your health, improve your vitality, and become the woman you were always meant to be.

The contents of these chapters are the result of thousands of hours of study, research, and personal experiences that stemmed from my own health struggles. My health challenges began around the age of eight and fluctuated through the years. The slow downward decline started with migraines, weight gain, and fatigue. By my late teens I was battling serious depression. In my early twenties I began to experience severe muscle tension and started seeing chiropractors and physical therapists but noticed no improvement. I rallied through my mid-twenties with mediocre health but no diagnosis of any problem. However, at the age of 26, after an exceptionally stressful period in my life, my doctor discovered a large cyst on my ovary. Following the subsequent surgery and removal, things became progressively worse.

I began to experience unrelenting depression, fatigue, brain fog, lack of concentration, anxiety, and hormone imbalances. In spite of these setbacks, I was eventually blessed with two healthy baby girls born three years apart. The trade-off was two nine-month periods of constant nausea, inability to cope or make decisions, bodily pains, and migraines. Each nine month period was followed by years of postpartum depression.

At the age of 35 I was diagnosed with thyroid cancer and had a complete thyroidectomy. Fortunately, the doctor found the cancer early and I made a full recovery. A year later another doctor discovered elevated levels of mercury and lead in my blood, also known as heavy metal toxicity.

Through my earlier physical pains and setbacks I held on to my belief in God, and my belief that there was a reason for all things. But after my second pregnancy, I could no longer tolerate the suffering and I turned my heart away from God. I could not understand how a loving Father could allow such misery without heeding my need for help. Of all the pains endured, separation from God was the hardest. I became bitter, angry, and lost.

I went through a ten year period where I chose to isolate myself from other women because I did not feel like myself. I would attend work, church, and my children's school events but knew I was only going through the motions. There were periods of time where I was more able to function than others, but I never once believed that this was the way a woman was supposed to feel. I knew that for some reason my body was broken and I was determined to find out why.

Over the last decade I have seen dozens of doctors—both medically and holistically trained—and read countless sources of health information. I took notes and stockpiled knowledge whenever I could. On other days when I was able, I studied and searched volumes of information about everything from nutrition to brain chemistry, from emotional issues to cancer. And it was through this research that I began to see the complex connections and intertwined causes of today's health issues emerge. Once my body began to heal, I documented these causes and solutions with the hope of helping others.

I was determined to discover why the female body becomes sick and imbalanced and how to regain joy and vitality. I was on a mission to heal myself—with or without God's help. Luckily, He helped me in spite of myself, with trails of breadcrumbs and gentle blessings along the way.

I realize that there are many books available on women's health. If you are reading this, you are likely to have read others in your own personal journey. But this publication is a little different; the material presented here is meant to educate you on how to heal the body so you can regain your birthright of emotional, physical, and *spiritual* health. The body and the spirit rely on each other, and the knowledge of how to repair that connection when it has been broken is needed today more than ever.

I also realize that women, and especially mothers, are the

busiest people on the planet. They don't have time to look into all the latest health advice and often wonder which suggestions will actually improve their lives. I have sifted through volumes of information so you don't have to. I have included health advice, product recommendations, and supplement suggestions that have repeatedly healed others, as well as myself, and allowed them to function again.

It is my goal and heartfelt desire to help women get well and reconnect with their inner spirit. I firmly believe that healthy women are the foundation of strong families, thriving kids, happy marriages, and successful communities. I believe by supporting and healing women, they can then support and heal their spouses, children, and neighborhoods, and make amazing things happen.

We will cover many topics together. If will-power, discipline, or memory is a problem for you, I encourage you to reprint the pages that apply to your situation, or take notes in the margins and have someone you love help you pull this information together. When you make a plan for yourself and enlist someone else to help you stick to it, you will have a much greater chance of success.

I pray that this information helps you or someone you love to shorten their path back to health. From my own seemingly endless journey, I know it can be done. I send you love and compassion. But most of all I send you HOPE.

Chapter 1
IN THE BEGINNING…
Setting the Stage

We were put on this earth to fulfill the great measure of our potential. But having a broken body and a clouded mind disconnects us from our spiritual side, stifles our ability to feel, and prevents us from reaching that potential. Life should be fulfilling and rewarding. Life should feel worth living! When we restore our health and reconnect with our spirit, we can feel true joy again. We can live in the moment, full of love and with a passion for life. Most importantly, we are able to feel in touch with the universe and God when our broken vessel is restored.

The purpose of this book is to teach you how to heal your body so you can reconnect with your spirit. The information packed into the following pages will help you to combat depression, illness, hormonal imbalance, loneliness, and negative behaviors and regain your former health. The knowledge therein contains solid, history-proven methods on how to restore your health and vitality. This material holds true regardless of our similarities or differences in personal religious beliefs. But because of my personal health journey and spiritual background, I cannot deny the guidance and paths that led me to this knowledge. Nor can I remain silent about the forces that are working against us all.

To explain how this journey began, I need to set the stage. I was born and raised in Huntsville, Alabama, in the Seventies. My father was raised as a Methodist and my mother grew up in the Baptist faith but joined The Church of Jesus Christ of Latter-day Saints when I was still an infant.

I grew up with a Methodist father and a Mormon mother—both of whom were exceptionally good people. However, it was my mother who assumed the role of spiritual teacher and took me and my siblings to church every week. I was blessed to have two parents who cared about their children and gave them all they could. In return, I worked hard in school, went to church regularly, and tried to be a good kid. I was far from being a perfect daughter, but I honestly worked hard to respect the love and opportunities my parents had given me.

Because of the loving examples of my parents, I desired to learn more about God and His truth. From studying and applying many of the teachings held in the scriptures, I developed a strong belief in the words of Jesus Christ and in the prophets who testified of Him.

I believe in a loving Heavenly Father who gave all of us the opportunity to come to Earth and receive mortal bodies. I believe that in the beginning, long before we arrived here, we were happy and innocent spiritual children who knew nothing of discomfort, grief, temptation, or sadness. We understood that in order to grow we needed to receive a physical body and go through a mortal life. To never experience a human life or separation from God, would leave us unable to understand true joy, freedom of choice, or how amazing God truly is.

Our Heavenly Father presented a plan that would allow all his spirit children to obtain mortal bodies. We would get to experience pain, separation, and temptation. And yet, in time we would also obtain greater knowledge, understanding, and experience.

It is written that we shouted for joy at the unfolding of this plan[1]. God also prepared a way for us to return to him through a sinless third party. A Savior would suffer and atone for the sins of mankind that we might only need to have faith and repent to return unto the Father. Jesus Christ selflessly offered to fill this consecrated role, to make the necessary sacrifice and give all the glory unto the Father[2].

But there was some dissent. Lucifer presented a plan where we would all make it back effortlessly. He proposed simply that under his plan, no one would be allowed to sin and therefore all would return to Heavenly Father and the glory would go to Lucifer.

Heavenly Father knew that free agency was a crucial part of the plan of mortality and that it must be preserved for all. He denied Lucifer's plan and chose Christ to be the Savior of mankind. Lucifer (a.k.a. Satan, or the Adversary) was livid his proposal had been denied. He, along with his followers who wanted to remove free agency from God's plan, was cast down[3]. They were sent to earth but without mortal bodies.

Lucifer and his followers despise those of us who chose to follow God's plan of agency, for we have been given the gift of mortal bodies. They have been removed from the light of our Father and Christ and want only to inflict misery on those of us living on the earth. God knew we would need to be tempted in order to understand the difference between good and evil, and virtue and vice. With His infinite knowledge, Heavenly Father placed protection between us and them[4]: they can tempt us and give us ideas, but they cannot force us to act on the thoughts with which they influence us. Who we eventually become is entirely up to us and what we choose to believe.

Some people in the world today speak of these ideas to do evil as our Ego (or in Freud's case, the "id"), and indicate it lies within us and is part of us. What philosophers conveniently forget to consider is the power of a carefully placed suggestion. I believe the Ego they speak of is actually the human part of each one of us that is highly susceptible to temptations from the minions of Lucifer who want us to be miserable like they are.

The only power they have is to influence us with negative, selfish, wrong, and evil ideas. These thoughts take flight only when we allow them to sway our actions. By acting upon these negative impulses, we can certainly infuse them into our souls and become selfish and egotistical. However, our personal power lies in the ability to disbelieve and not act upon these ideas.

We are empowered when we realize *where* these negative ideas are coming from. It helps to know that these thoughts and ideas are not initially our own—they do not originate within us and we are not fundamentally bad people. Without this necessary opposition we could never learn and grow. **However, it is also helpful to realize that our inherent ability to fight against temptation and make wise choices is compromised when our bodies are unhealthy and our minds are imbalanced.**

I know this to be true because I learned it firsthand. After I succumbed to many lies and temptations I discovered books on the complex and subtle deceptions of the Adversary and recognized them instantly as what I had thought were my own thoughts. Looking back, I realized I had been completely duped by the Adversary at times, and had made terrible choices. This realization caused me great sadness.

For example, one of these events occurred while I attended college at Brigham Young University. For those of you unfamiliar with this school, BYU is not like most other universities. There is a strict Code of Conduct required by all who attend. Students agree to abstain from alcohol, smoking, drugs, and premarital sex and observe other guiding principles including honesty and integrity. All who attend agree to adhere to the rules. If you don't want to follow the guidelines, there are a plethora of other universities available to the college-bound student. For me, I wanted very much to attend BYU. I knew I needed to avoid the distractions that commonly occur at other learning institutions and I wanted to be surrounded by other people who desired the same.

Unfortunately, once I got settled for my first semester, I felt very different from other students. I had always had lots of friends in Alabama but felt very out of place at BYU. It was likely because of poor choices made during my high school years. I chose to be friends with a rough crowd and kept one foot in the world and one foot in church. I made good grades and attended seminary, but there weren't many kids to hang out with who held to the high standards that I had been taught. During high school, I was drawn to the "cool crowd" and was curious about all the substances I had been told to stay away from. Even though I knew the gospel of Christ was true and I wanted to be a part of it, I loved people and didn't want to have to isolate myself to avoid negative influences.

Fortunately, I humbled myself, repented and was able to apply and attend BYU, but didn't realize my former bad habits would make adjusting to life at college so much harder. What I didn't understand was that every moment you spend doing not-so-great things affects your body and spirit. It is actually written on your countenance and others can see and sense it.

I had a friend from my freshman BYU dorm tell me that many of the girls on my floor were scared of me when they first met me. How sad! I had no idea that spending years having "fun" in ways that were not conducive to keeping the Spirit of God would affect my heart and what it perceived as fun in the future. Ice blocking, going for ice cream at the Creamery, and planning harmless pranks on boys seemed like complete childishness to me. I wanted to go to parties and socialize with people who were more experienced in the ways of the world. The purity of Mormon students often left me feeling like I was surrounded by children and I longed for a more complex crowd to hang out with.

I also didn't realize that because of my genetic make-up and previous bad habits, I had way too many toxins in my physical body. While I was out partying, I was not only polluting my spirit, but my body as well. Normally, a person could recover from what I had done and have no physical ramifications. However in my weakened body, the toxins and stress I put on my liver literally caused me to become sick and depressed. How I learned this, years later, is explained more in the chapter titled "Toxicity and Your Genetic Make-up."

I obeyed all the rules outlined in the Code of Conduct for my first year, went to church, served in my church callings (volunteer positions) and studied the scriptures. I learned a lot, and was greatly humbled. But I also felt out of place and disconnected. By the second semester of my sophomore year, I had become so desperate that I sought out people and places that would help me escape from my pain and, of course, found some. I bet if you've ever gone looking for trouble you found it easier than you left it. I desperately wanted the mental pain to stop but thought it was *my own desires* that were causing my problems. I didn't realize I was experiencing a classic case of depression—not only from my previous abuses on my body but also from a lack of Vitamin D and heavy metal toxicity.

Please listen and share this message: Satan will use whatever lies he can to break you down. For me, he worked on my deep sense of inward guilt that I could not seem to obey the Word of Wisdom (a guideline asking Mormons to avoid alcohol, tobacco, coffee and tea, and use moderation in all things), that I would never fit in as a member of the Church, and that I was especially unfit to attend a university that I perceived to be full of such pure, obedient people. Some examples of negative thoughts that entered my mind were:

- You obviously need to leave BYU and let someone more worthy take your place. Lots of people want to be there. You shouldn't be taking up a spot if you can't honor the Code of Conduct—and you can't seem to keep it together.
- If you don't feel like you belong here now, why would you ever feel at home with these people in heaven? You would surely feel out of place there, too. Why are you working so hard to arrive at a place where you will never belong?
- If you know the gospel of Christ is true then you are obviously just not strong enough to live it fully. You should give up and go to school where all your old friends are and leave the church. It will be better for everyone for you to just leave.

Many miraculous events occurred soon thereafter that allowed me to change my heart and mind and stay at BYU. These events included my mother being inspired to pray for me insistently even though she didn't know why; two bishops intervening on my behalf; and a professor, who was also a professional counselor, taking me under his wing and counseling me for an hour each week—for free—for an entire semester. Much humble gratitude goes to these people. But through that entire experience, I never realized I was clinically depressed.

Depression is diagnosed and understood much better

today, but I believe there are rapidly increasing numbers of people who suffer from undiagnosed nutritional deficiencies, borderline mental issues, and feelings of disconnection and hopelessness. These problems affect our ability to feel connected to God. Furthermore, life decisions made by those suffering from poor mental and physical health affect lives and families for generations.

Several years later I was told I should read a book called *Putting on the Armor of God* by Steven A. Cramer. I was at another low point and seeking for spiritual help and guidance. This book was a huge eye-opener for me. The content goes through the fall of Lucifer and how he became Satan, the "Father of all Lies." It reveals the history, methods, and tactical maneuvers of the Adversary as he and his minions try to bring down the children of men.

Make no mistake; we are at war *every day*. The only problem is that most of us don't even realize it! Once you understand your enemy, you can arm yourself with the armor of God and be prepared for any attack. I highly recommend this book. Its contents are truly inspired and it changed my view on everyday human life and the importance of the gospel of Jesus Christ.

By reading Steven Cramer's book, I found example after example of the EXACT negative thoughts I had had when I nearly left BYU. I had thought they were MY thoughts and thus, true for me. It turns out I had been a victim of some very cruel, debilitating, and untrue ideas. And these ideas weren't original or unique—they had been used for millennia. I felt foolish and as if I should have known better.

I became really angry when I realized I had been kicked when I was already down. There is something about anyone being bullied or taken advantage of when they desperately need support and assistance that makes me fuming mad. When it happens, I dig in my heels and won't give in to the abuser—no matter what.

My dad says stubbornness runs in our family. All I know is, whether it's me or someone else, when I see someone being bullied in any way I stand up and fight for them. Being kicked when you are down is Satan's most cowardly tactic, and as long as I have a voice, I will fight against it.

Today, more and more women are experiencing poor health, infertility, and depression. It is becoming an epidemic. As women succumb to these issues, spouses' and children's lives are being damaged in the process. Many of the health issues women have today are influenced by overzealous media proclamations of poorly executed scientific studies—studies which seem to have been influenced by the Adversary. These mistruths cause confusion that leads many to poor health and despair.

I believe it is very important for women to understand who and what is attacking their health and happiness. In this book, I will reveal not only the processes necessary to recover your health, but also the forces that are working against you.

Now that you understand the spiritual tone and beliefs this book is built upon, let's get started.

Chapter 2

THE DRIVER:

The Daily Race Between Mind and Spirit

If you think of your body as a car, you'll realize there can be two drivers vying for control: your mind and your spirit. To clarify, in this chapter, the spirit (lowercase) means *your* spirit, not The Spirit—as in The Spirit of God or The Spirit of the Holy Ghost. Your spirit is the entity that wants to connect with The Spirit—when connected, happiness flows. What we need to do more often as humans is let our spirits guide us, and put our minds in the backseat.

The mind is a mediocre driver at best. If you equate it to the "natural man," the mind is subject to carnal desires, and is sensual and devilish[5]. The mind at its worst cuts off other drivers, speeds excessively, never allows anyone to get in front of it, and makes life miserable for everyone in proximity. Even more concerning, an unbalanced, stressed mind causes horrible accidents that create sadness and misery for everyone involved.

The spirit is a much better driver. It knows exactly where to go and exactly when to get there. The spirit is never anxious or stressed. Unlike the selfish mind, the spirit allows others to merge into traffic and considers the bigger picture. The spirit knows all because it naturally connects to The Spirit. Our spirits willingly follow loving commands from our Heavenly Father who guides us back to the ultimate destination—His presence.

Let's be honest—when the coin is flipped each day that decides who gets to drive, the mind usually wins. The mind is our default driver where the spirit has to be invited. Unfortunately, we often speed along on cruise control with the mind at the wheel—the spirit patiently sitting in the backseat awaiting a long-overdue turn. In fact, the sad truth is that for most people, the mind always wins—they don't realize they have a choice.

Even for those of us who are aware of this choice, we wake up to an alarm and then rush to get to school or work or prepare others to do so. If we are wise, we will get up a little earlier to say prayers and read scriptures in order to reconnect our spirit to God's. Unfortunately, tiredness often wins out and prayers don't get said—or if they do, it is done hurriedly and without proper attention. Satan rejoices and then plans his attack for the next day, so we will be too tired, too stressed, and too busy to pray. Satan knows he has great opportunity to influence your mind when it is driving, but zero chance to influence your spirit driver when connected to The Spirit.

For many years, my poor mental and physical health affected my spirit's opportunities to drive. I was so angry at what felt like heavenly neglect throughout my second pregnancy that I could not pray. My first pregnancy was incredibly difficult. I had nausea, pain, mental stress, and sadness the entire time. It became so overwhelming that I finally agreed to take anti-depressants the month before my first child was born. After the delivery, I recovered somewhat in the next few months but felt like a zombie. My

OB suggested an IUD for birth control at nine weeks postpartum, so I agreed. I gained 40 pounds over the next nine months. I was not well. I chalked it up to recovering from a difficult pregnancy, but my body was completely out of whack. I felt overwhelmed, emotional, and completely unlike my normal self.

I had been taught that God wants his spirit children to be born into strong families on earth. Accordingly, my mind decided that my first pregnancy must have been hard because it was a girl. I just *knew* that my second child would be a boy and that the pregnancy would be easier. My mind told me that God would not have me endure a second experience just like the first, or else there would be no more children for us. As it turns out, my mind was wrong on all counts.

My second pregnancy was another seemingly unending bout of nausea, pain, depression, insomnia, and inability to cope or function. I liken it to fingernails on a chalkboard—for nine months. But this time, I also had zero ability to feel The Spirit. This time, I knew exactly how bad it was going to get and I couldn't even utter a prayer for help. I was so physically and spiritually broken that I would rather not ask than risk the chance of my prayer going unanswered and the lack of help completely severing my relationship with God.

In addition, despite the severe misery, every time I would go in for monthly check-ups, all my blood numbers, blood pressure, and sugar levels were just fine. I was afraid of being labeled as a patient who made up symptoms for attention. There was zero indication that I was enduring any stress or pain according to the limited monthly lab tests. I was very glad the baby was fine, but I longed for help in the form of some kind of diagnosis. I was too sick to think through my options for help. I just knew I had to buckle down and endure whatever was going on for the sake of the baby.

I knew from past personal experiences that most doctors do not know how to diagnose someone without lab tests showing something being specifically wrong. When you're pregnant, it's even harder to diagnose a problem without any lab markers. Doctors are also understandably hesitant to prescribe anything to a pregnant woman without absolute necessity. So I didn't tell my doctor about the extent of my misery.

I knew from my first pregnancy that he would simply prescribe me some supposedly "fetus-friendly" anti-depressant. I had already decided I would not get on medications without knowing what was wrong because I didn't want them to negatively impact my child's present state or future one. If all my markers were fine, I could only assume the baby was progressing normally, and I was just really lousy at being pregnant. I just held on and tried to get through each tortuous day. Time was not my friend. Each minute felt like an hour, each hour like a day. The nausea was unrelenting and the depression did not yield.

By the end of the pregnancy I was at the end of my rope. I had a scheduled C-section (my first daughter was also a C-section) so I could mentally hold on until that moment. After the baby arrived, blessedly healthy, I felt better immediately. The nausea was gone instantly, as well as the headaches, and physical pain.

But I was not well overall—I felt as if I had post-traumatic stress disorder. I felt as if I had been beaten and tortured for months as a prisoner of war. I did not feel as if I were supported and helped by the Savior through the horrors of those months. I felt neglected, abused, and beaten down. I understood why men come back from war and never pray again—and my heart broke at the understanding. Reading the "Footprints in the Sand" poem where Jesus carries the man during the hardest parts of his life would make me angry. Before, I had always believed the truth in that poem. But where was Jesus when I needed him most? Even if I had been unable to ask, wouldn't He help a child in need who was too sick to pray?

My stubborn nature would never allow an abuser to stay in my life, and I decided God would be no different. Make no mistake; neglect is just as bad as abuse—and in some cases, worse. What I perceived as Godly neglect caused me great pain and anger. I had made difficult sacrifices in my life to align my life choices with His teachings. I had forgone friends, dreams, and bad influences to know God. I had repented when I made mistakes. I had read my scriptures, prayed, and done volunteer work in my church when given the opportunity.

It was my understanding that God would never give us more than we could handle. But my two pregnancies and the aftermath of each were way more than my mind could bear. So I shut my heart from God.

In essence, I hogtied my spirit and shoved it in the backseat. I'm pretty sure I duct taped my spirit's mouth as well because it was pretty quiet back there. For years I suffered through each day, watching and waiting for some kind of easing of the physical, mental, and spiritual pain. I was not living—I was just barely getting by. In my stubbornness and state of mind-driven self-protection, there was no way my spirit was going to tell me anything other than what my mind had decided: that God had turned his back on me when I needed Him the most. It took years for me to come around and revisit that decision.

My complete refusal to allow God in my life made an already sickly life an even sadder one. **With 20/20 hindsight, I now know that my mind was affected by imbalanced hormones, toxicity, and severe malnutrition.** My spirit couldn't break through to my broken brain. Like a child who believes he or she is unlovable because of a divorce or abuse, I clung stubbornly to an untrue belief created from poor information. It was a sad, lonely, and painful experience—and one I hope that more women will be able to avoid.

From this experience, I realized that no one can change your thoughts for you. You have complete control over your beliefs and actions. However, if you suffer from mental and physical imbalances and illness, the cards are most certainly stacked against you. In order for you to have a fighting chance in this world, you need to be physically and mentally strong. If you suffer from depression, illness, mental issues, or hormone problems, I would like you to climb into the backseat and keep reading. Let me drive you for a while. We are headed for a place of hope and healing.

Chapter 3

THE TEETH MYSTERY:

Discovering the Four Pillars of Good Health

I love people's hands. I have a tendency to notice the shape and size of the palms, the lengths of the fingers, and the shape of people's fingernails. For the longest time (before brain fog set in and my memory clouded), I even had stored in my mind a recollection of the hands of my friends and co-workers. Once I admitted this to a group of co-workers who immediately grilled me to describe each of their hands. Once I was done, they were a little shocked at the accuracy. I can't explain it. I just love hands.

But there is one thing I love even more than hands, and that's teeth. I am a sucker for a beautiful smile. I have to admit that a great smile was magnetizing to me while looking for Mr. Right. For a long time I wasn't sure where my obsession came from. But then I had an epiphany. As a little child, I remember my mother telling me how both she and Dad had been blessed with good teeth. Neither of them had ever needed braces. She'd always been very grateful for her healthy, straight teeth and hoped all three of us children would inherit that trait. Luckily, my brother and sister never needed braces. Then there was me.

Nothing in life quite compares with those months of pain, awkwardness, and misery while you are afflicted with a mouth full of metal. Add to that an already unfortunate adolescent skin issue. Then add a weight problem, and the condition was complete: soul-crushing, self-esteem annihilating female adolescence. The one thing I had going for me at the end of those painful months, when the metal was removed, was a pretty decent smile. For the first time I began to get compliments on something. That's when my obsession with teeth began.

Five years later I got to attend the London Study Abroad program through BYU. Our group was in York, England, going through the Jorvik Viking Museum when I spotted it: a skull with unbelievably perfect teeth. We are talking about 5 years of braces, tooth shaping, and perfect whitening kind-of-teeth. I was drawn to it like a moth to a flame. I read the placard underneath the skull and my jaw dropped: Viking Skull, estimated circa 866-1066 A.D.

I was stunned.

They didn't even have braces back then! How could this Viking have had such a perfect set of teeth? This experience undeniably seared itself into my teeth-loving brain. I pondered it over time and time again. It wasn't until years later that the answer of how this Viking won the teeth-lottery presented itself to me.

The Dental Anthropologist

Fast forward 12 years during which I suffered through three surgeries, two devastatingly difficult pregnancies, a bout with cancer, and too many other health problems to count. I was desperately trying to reclaim my health and had started forcing myself to learn how to cook. (It's amazing how long you can get by on a few basic dishes and lots of take-out.) Eventually I stumbled upon *Nourishing Traditions* by Sally Fallon. I highly recommend this book for its well-researched nutrition knowledge and cooking advice. From this book, I learned a great deal about fermentation, preparing grains for the human body, and the place organ meats should and could have in our diets. Her teaching points were absolutely new to me. But the most eye-opening thing I learned from this book was about the work of Dr. Weston Price.

Dr. Weston Price was a dentist from Ohio who began to notice a general deterioration of his patients' physical and dental health in the 1930's. He began to wonder what was causing the decline. He knew his patients needed advice on how to protect and strengthen their teeth but he didn't know the answers. Dr. Price devised a plan and proceeded to travel around the globe studying tribal peoples' lifestyles and eating habits to see how these affected their teeth. What he discovered was amazing.

"Dr. Price found fourteen primitive groups—from isolated Irish and Swiss, from Eskimos to Africans—in which almost every member of the tribe or village enjoyed superb health. They were free of chronic disease, dental decay and mental illness; they were strong, sturdy and attractive; and they produced healthy children with ease, generation after generation.

Dr. Price had many opportunities to compare these healthy so-called "primitives" with members of the same racial group who had become "civilized" and were living on the products of the industrial revolution—refined grains, canned foods, pasteurized milk and sugar. In these peoples, he found rampant tooth decay, infectious disease, degenerative illness and infertility. Children born to traditional peoples who had adopted the industrialized diet had crowded and crooked teeth, narrowed faces, deformities of bone structure and susceptibility to every sort of medical problem. Studies too numerous to count have confirmed Dr. Price's observations that the so-called civilized diet, particularly the Western diet of refined carbohydrates and devitalized fats and oils, spoils our God-given genetic inheritance of physical perfection and vibrant health.[6]

There was the answer: beautiful teeth require beautiful nutrition. Not the 1970's trans-fat fried-everything-washed-down-with-a-soda diet I grew up on. I read Sally's book from cover to cover, which I highly recommend you do as well. I cannot possibly articulate the beauty of soaked grains and nuts, or the essence of a great fermented dish to the same degree of detail that she provided. Yet her book started me on more of my own research, and I soon realized that people living in cultures that had some form of fermented foods in their diet, ate good fats, and had no sugar or processed grains led amazingly healthy lives. These people were free of obesity, depression, and cancer. They were active their entire lives and were free of dementia. The majority lived to ripe old ages and died in their sleep.

Dr. Price analyzed the diets of these primitive peoples and found they had at least **four** times the calcium and minerals and at least **ten** times the fat-soluble vitamins from animal foods such as butter, fish, eggs, shellfish, and organ meats as compared to our modern-day diets. I suddenly realized how compromised our Western diet really is—and how our children's health would continue to deteriorate with every mother who was too busy to prepare meals or who had never been properly taught how and what to cook.

So let's think for a minute. If it was your goal to break down the entire human population into a society of sick, hormonally-imbalanced, depressed, rage-filled, infertile masses, where would you start? What group of people would affect generations to come, thus accelerating your misery-inducing plan? You would probably start with the nurturers, care-givers, and cooks of the family—or, in other words, women.

I've got news for you. The Adversary has already thought this one out—and it is working. In fact, after malnourishing the masses he knows that if you throw three more ingredients into the mix, you could have an almost-perfect storm of disease within the human body. This holds especially true for the female body since the delicate nature of the hormonal cascade within women makes us more vulnerable to any attack.

There were three more things these primal groups were blessed to avoid that we are not, and how our bodies handle these elements can mean the difference between life and death.

The First Element: Toxins

In our modern world we sleep on sheets washed with chemicals, arise to brush our teeth and clean our bodies with parabens and phthalates, and then eat a breakfast of genetically-modified, processed cereal grains, and complete the meal with some pesticide-covered fruit. Maybe if you're uber-healthy you try to get in a run or bike ride next to vehicles spewing toxic exhaust fumes. Good Morning!

We literally bombard ourselves with—or we are bombarded by—multiple toxin-sources every single day. Most of us don't even think about it. Our bodies are truly amazing in their ability to remove toxins from our cells. After researching this topic, I am surprised more of us don't have bigger health problems.

Fortunately, the human body has several mechanisms to help us get rid of the stuff we don't want around:

- The skin
- The liver
- The lymph system
- The kidneys
- The colon

When all of these systems are working properly, the body does a pretty good job of detoxifying itself. But what happens when one of the systems fails, gets overloaded, or doesn't get the support it needs to function properly? Big problems, that's what happens. Unfortunately, today we have such a constant barrage of toxins coming our way that there's literally no time for our systems to rest. They have to work at full-capacity every single day just to keep up.

What are some of the ways toxicity shows up in humans? Here are just a few: fatigue, gall stones, migraines, depression, allergies, cancer, insomnia, and infertility. Imagine being free of all of these things. What an amazing thought!

I'm not trying to be the bearer of unbearable news. There are many things we can do to avoid or assist in accelerating the exit of toxins. I'm going to dive into them in more detail in a future chapter. But for now just know that toxicity is a very real problem and we need to do all we can to support our bodies in this never-ending job.

The Second Element: Stress

Women today are under ever increasing amounts of stress. We occupy many roles every day: mother, wife, daughter, sister, friend, business owner, employee, church-volunteer, school-volunteer, chauffeur, chef, family nutritionist, cheerleader, problem solver, and birthday party planner, among others. We care deeply about our family, friends, and their well-being and are constantly concerned on their behalf.

Tribal people may not have access to movies, cars, and pharmacies, but I'm betting they may have less self-inflicted stress in their lives as a bonus. How is it that we live lives so very busy that we don't even have time to say a prayer—or have a spare second to act upon a spiritual prompting?

When we ask ourselves whose plan excessive busyness and stress advances I think we will all agree that it is not God's.

The constant bombardment of toxins we experience every day can still pale in comparison to the amount of stress we inflict—or have inflicted—upon ourselves as we strive to live what we hope are virtuous, Christ-centered lives.

> An old friend of mine jokingly warned me once to never pray for patience or humility because life would be sure to dish up plenty of both all on its own. He was so right.

I remember a woman who gave a presentation on stress in Relief Society (the women's class in my church) many years ago. She had just moved to our area from another state, had a husband who traveled, and five children ranging from toddlers to teenagers. As an object lesson she pulled out a huge poster board with lists (in very small print) of all the things she had to do and all the things that were causing her stress.

I promise you, she read off that poster board for over 5 minutes. She had a *lot* of things on her plate. At that time I was married but didn't have children yet. I was completely overwhelmed by her long list and felt sorry that I didn't better know how to help her. Since then, I have learned to be careful what I wish for (ha ha). Today I know all too well what she felt like that day and wish I could have served her better back then.

The Third Element: Isolation

The peoples Dr. Price studied were not only well-nourished, but well-connected. These tribes and groups had to work together out of necessity. People knew each other and which children belonged to each family. Mothers and grandmothers kept an eye out for all the children, not just their own. As advancements in technology, travel, and education have allowed more people to relocate, the kind of community Dr. Price documented is now a rarity.

Children grow up and often move to a new location because of a job opportunity. Over time, extended families rarely live in the same area. People have to try to create new social bonds each time they move. Some people are gifted in this area while others are not.

In current-day cities, people rarely know their neighbors and a lack of community is the inevitable result. Humans were not meant to live in isolation. When a sense of connectedness exists, humans thrive. Stress is reduced, communication increases, and lifespans lengthen. Without it, people turn to other distractions including virtual worlds, TV programs, gaming, addiction, and crime. All of these are poor substitutions for human interaction and a sense of belonging.

Nutrition, toxin removal, stress management, and a sense of community are the four pillars of a healthy body. Any one of these being compromised can knock our lives off balance. I hope to arm you with the knowledge you need to assist your body in the healing process so you can regain your own sense of balance. I also hope to give you encouragement and support. You are beloved by your Heavenly Father and you are not forgotten—even if you are only hanging on by "the skin of your teeth."

Chapter 4
MENTAL ILLNESS AND YOUR TWO BRAINS

Illness. Think for a minute about what that word means to you. Obviously, it's the opposite of *wellness.* And it isn't limited to the body—just as there is physical illness, there is also mental illness. And while you would never think to blame someone for her bone cancer or shingles or multiple sclerosis, you'd be shocked at how often people get blamed for their depression or anxiety or paranoia.

I want to open a dialogue among women that will help remove the stigma and shame associated with having a mental illness. I'm not coming at this from a removed, clinical point of view. I personally struggled through years of sadness, depression, anxiety, and paranoia—and I did the very best I could to keep it all a secret. I felt incredibly isolated and alone, but I didn't dare let others know about my "problems." I didn't want their pity. Even worse, I'd seen too many people who were shunned and mistreated as a result of problems like mine, and I didn't want to end up even more isolated. I knew I wasn't healthy, but I didn't know how to fix it. In fact, I didn't know if it *could* be fixed.

Right up front, it's important to understand that mental illness is not the fault of the afflicted person. If you are struggling with mental issues, it's not because you're not positive enough, not strong enough, not prayerful enough, not smart enough, or not motivated enough to get well. In this chapter we will connect the dots between your body's two brains and how they affect each other. Once you understand some of the causes of mental illness, you will have the power to take control of your own well-being. You may find that you have more power to heal yourself than you ever thought possible.

Fortunately for those who suffer today, societal attitudes have become more accepting towards mental illness. And while there is still much room for improvement, it was quite common a generation ago to think of mental illness as a weakness or shortcoming. Consider also, that for the generation before our parents' it was unspeakable—even shameful—to have a nervous breakdown or admit any sort of mental "imbalance," and we realize that perceptions have certainly shifted.

Just two generations ago, no one even *talked* about depression. But if you're like most people today, you know of at least one case of depression, anxiety, or attention deficit disorder within your circle of acquaintances. It may even be you who suffers from bipolar disorder, schizophrenia, or one of the many other types of mental illness.

Depression seems to be an increasingly common ailment today, particularly in the state of Utah. I have lost count of the number of my friends who are on anti-depressants. Utah doctors prescribe more anti-depressants than any other state in the country[7]. And I have no doubt many of the rest of the population are self-medicating with alcohol and illicit drugs.

Why are we all so sad? What is making us unwell?

There *is* an answer—and, better yet, there are solutions. What you're about to read will help you start to understand the causes and cures.

As mentioned, I struggled with mental issues for years, and I felt painfully isolated and alone. Believe me when I say that was a huge change from my normal personality. I love people and have been blessed in the past to have many close friends. But during that time, I felt like an outsider, even when I was surrounded by others—even at my own daughter's birthday party. My most common prayer during that time was, "Please, give me my brain back." I had a hard time remembering things. I felt foggy-headed most of the time. I couldn't carry on conversations like I'd always been able to. I used to intuitively know how to put people at ease and make them laugh—but while I was ill, I could scarcely think of a topic to discuss, let alone harness the vocabulary needed to express my thoughts. I was humiliated at the change in my personality and intellect. To say it was humbling is putting it mildly. I felt *extreme* mental and social anxiety every single day for more than a decade.

I'm going to testify about something very important to you, because I learned it from firsthand experience. If you're struggling with mental issues like I was, the Adversary wants you to think that you're weak and pathetic—and that your problems are entirely your fault. He wants you to remain miserable and hopeless. He doesn't want you to know that you are being stealthily assaulted from all sides. He doesn't want you to know there is a solution to your problem.

Contrast that to your Heavenly Father, who loves you beyond understanding. He adores you and is aware of your pain. He is also very aware of Satan's attack. He allows it only because every bit of suffering we endure will make us stronger. But there comes a time when you've learned all you can from a trial and it's time to move forward. Enough is enough. If you are reading this, it's time for you to learn how to fight back and understand how to win—and I know that feeling, because I finally reached that point myself.

I decided I needed to address some unresolved issues from my past and began to search for a psychologist. I was referred to a great counselor who helped me understand many earlier hurtful experiences and how to work through them. The problem was that I knew I was feeling pain from past experiences far too intensely. These emotions would rise to the surface and linger for days. I instinctively knew something was wrong *physically* that was keeping me from healing *emotionally*.

As I researched more and more articles, books, and blogs on female health I avidly looked for information on the brain. Then, I found a book that changed my life: *The Ultramind Solution* by Dr. Mark Hyman. Dr. Hyman is a pioneer in the fight to educate people on *functional medicine*, the practice of looking at the body as a whole instead of considering only individual symptoms. For example, if you had intestinal pains, your primary care physician would probably refer you to a gastroenterologist. But let's say the gastroenterologist diagnosed your problem as endometriosis and then referred you to a gynecologist. Would the two doctors work together? Not likely in today's medical system.

Now look at how it works under the theory of functional medicine. Your physician would do a full examination of your entire body, run a complete blood panel and then consider all your symptoms, regardless of whether they seem related. With an accurate picture of what is going on in your entire body, your physician would then work to solve the problem at the source instead of simply addressing the end result of the illness, performing surgery or prescribing pharmaceuticals to manage your symptoms.

From reading Dr. Hyman's work, and many other sources on brain health, I began to see a pattern emerge. Brain health simply requires the proper balance of brain chemicals and raw materials for maintenance.

So what affects this brain chemistry balance at the source?

The answer is so simple it's astounding. Pure and simple, it's the *gut*. And odd as it may seem, the gut functions much like your brain.

That's Right: You Have Two Brains

In 2005, I accompanied my husband on a work reward trip to Cabo San Lucas. I'd never been there and was excited to go with some of my husband's colleagues and their wives. Our hotel was beautiful and the sunsets were breathtaking. We enjoyed amazing food and events planned by the company. Everyone was having a wonderful time—until "Montezuma's revenge" was unleashed.

The third night of our stay, our group went to a dinner downtown. The food was great, and we didn't think twice about eating it. Unfortunately, the next day several of us *wished* we had thought twice. I began re-experiencing the nausea I had dealt with during my pregnancies. But just as it had been during my pregnancies, I rarely threw up or had diarrhea—I just had continuous nonstop misery. It was over a week before I felt somewhat normal again.

During that episode I got to learn again how problems with your intestines affect your mind. Throughout this stint of Montezuma's revenge—just as during my pregnancies—I felt depressed, overwhelmed, sad, irritated, and believed the sun would never shine again. Later, as I studied more about the connection between the brain and the intestines, I began to understand there is a much stronger connection between the two than most people realize. In fact, the intestines affect the brain much more than the brain affects the intestines, despite what you may believe about a "nervous stomach."

In some cultures, the gut is referred to as the second brain. Take a look at why this is true. You've heard the phrase "gut instinct"—and there's a reason why you feel things in your gut. The gut has several layers in order to digest, move, and protect the body from outside substances. One of these layers is composed of nervous system cells. These nerves orchestrate digestion and the constant advancement of food along the intestinal tract. If they were isolated and joined together they would form a clump of neurons larger than the brain in your head. The brain in the gut drives your feelings and intuition by electrical signals created from these nervous tissue cells. Translation: you must have a healthy intestinal system to feel peaceful, balanced, and intuitive[8].

The other reason your gut is your second brain is because it produces the lion's share of neurotransmitters required by your body. For example, 90% of the brain chemical serotonin is produced there from the food you eat. That's right—most of this "brain chemical" is not manufactured in your brain at all, but in your gut. Serotonin is then delivered to the brain where it gives you a happy, calm feeling.

If you already realize that what you eat affects your moods, you're ahead of the game—but you may not realize just *how much* food is affecting your brain. It can make you happy and elated (sugary carbs or chocolate, anyone?) or severely depressed, anxious, paranoid, or foggy-headed (especially if you have food sensitivities or allergies). And it can do this in a matter of minutes—sometimes even less. This result can be so powerful that it can make you feel like you are out of control.

Those carbohydrate cravings you have in the afternoon? That may be your body telling you it wants more serotonin. It might even come from invaders in your intestines clamoring for more sugar. That craving for chocolate during your monthly cycle is a similar situation created from imbalanced brain chemistry and hormones.

I have a dear friend that I've known since we were toddlers, whom we will call Bella. In her thirties Bella realized she was an alcoholic, and with her family's help and support, she checked into rehab. The first thing the clinic did was give her an antidepressant. Apparently the withdrawal effects are much better managed when the brain is getting another form of chemical support. The rehab center had also learned that patients had far fewer relapses while on antidepressants. Could this indicate that addictions are simply the body's response to a deficiency in neurotransmitters for the brain?

I noticed that when I took the antidepressant Buproprion (also known as Wellbutrin), I didn't feel a constant need to eat carbohydrates. In fact, I ate less food without even trying and lost about ten pounds. This was a unique event for me. Ever since the age of eight, I'd had a very hard time feeling full and was overweight most of my life. I believe now that my brain chemistry was imbalanced. My brain was so desperately in need of a boost in brain chemicals that it sent out almost constant hunger signals. Bella may be an alcoholic, but I am a carb-oholic without question.

Problems in your gut lead to problems everywhere else in your body. This is especially true for the delicate balance in our brains. It is no wonder that today women everywhere are fighting with depression and other brain disorders.

Now that you know *where* the problem originates. It's time to look at the *sources* of the problem—and prepare to be surprised.

What Could Possibly Be Wrong?

I will go into greater detail in subsequent chapters—but in a nutshell, there are three sources to every problem with the gut and brain, which just happen to be some of the same causes of illness mentioned earlier:

1. Lack of proper vitamins, minerals, or good bacteria—all of which are needed for the body to function normally, avoid/control inflammation, and defend itself from unwanted invaders
2. Toxicity
3. Stress

These three problems manifest themselves in many different ways *but they all start in the gut.*

Let's consider some examples. You probably haven't given much thought to the silver-colored fillings in your teeth. But did you know that the mercury in amalgam tooth fillings ends up in trace amounts in the intestines? Mercury has been proven to prevent the absorption of B vitamins through the gut. A deficiency in B vitamins is a known cause of depression[9] [10]. You may have never linked those childhood cavities with your feelings of sadness.

Another common problem occurs when you take antibiotics, eat too much sugar, or don't eat enough foods rich in fiber. When any of those happen, candida fungi in our intestines grow rapidly and crowd out the good bacteria in your gut. The result? The good bacteria can no longer assimilate nutrients to our body's tissues.

That's not all—and here's where the toxicity comes in. The candida produce noxious toxins that overwhelm your immune system and travel to your organs—including your brain—causing all kinds of havoc along the way.

Now factor in stress. It's related to the gut as well: 70 percent of the body's immune forces reside in the intestines. Unrelenting, persistent stress affects the contents of the gut, eventually breaking down our immune systems. The truth is that your body can handle enormous amounts of stress if it has the raw materials (vitamins, minerals, and healthy fats) needed for the fight at its disposal. You'll learn a lot more about that in a later chapter.

The digestive tract is a highly complex machine that, when it works properly, requires no thought at all. We usually only pay attention when pain or discomfort forces the issue. Unfortunately, more and more people are having pains and discomforts of all kinds. Reported cases of irritable bowel syndrome, Crohn's disease, Celiac disease, diverticulitis, intestinal and colon cancer are on the rise. All these illnesses are the end result of some sort of imbalance or assault upon the intestinal tract.

Only rarely is anyone born with these diseases; they almost always occur gradually over time. So what are we doing that would set us up for years of pain and suffering and perhaps shorten our lives?

It's all in what we eat—or in some cases, what we no longer consume.

Take a look at the average American diet. Most people in the United States eat large quantities of bread, cheese, corn, sugar, processed food, and industrially raised animal proteins with a salad here and there thrown in for good measure. Many of these foods have been altered from their original source and covered in pesticides—but this fact remains unknown by the majority of the population. And it's not just *what* we eat but *how* we eat—gulping down our food as we hurry to work, the next child's activity, or some other appointment.

Your body was not designed to eat that kind of diet, and was certainly not designed to eat on the run. You need lots of natural fiber; vegetables grown in mineral-rich soil; clean, humanely raised animal protein; a good amount of healthy fats; and probiotic-rich foods. You need those things *every day*. And you need to eat all that good food in a calm, relaxed environment. Do you know anyone who gets anywhere near enough of these foods— and who eats in that kind of environment?

What I've shared is just the tip of the iceberg. In the next chapters, I'll discuss dietary concerns in great detail. You'll learn how our sources of nutrients have been depleted, hybridized, and genetically altered—and how you can compensate. You will also learn a lot more about the inner workings of your gut and how to keep it healthy. You'll find out how caring for your second brain dramatically improves the well-being of your other brain.

Information is power—when you know why you are sad, sick, and depressed you'll have the knowledge you need to change your life and reclaim your connection to God. Here's to your personal journey back!

Chapter 5
INTOLERANCE AND SENSITIVITY:

How to Protect Yourself from Unknown Dangers

Intolerance and sensitivity. No, I'm not talking about a Jane Austen novel; I'm talking about food. Food intolerances and sensitivities are on the rise and no one is immune. More and more people struggle through the day with no energy, reduced mental capacity, pain and tension, and don't even realize that the cause is what is on their plate. It took me years to pinpoint the causes of my pain and suffering when all I needed to do was look down and notice what was on my fork.

Let's discuss why this is becoming more pervasive and what you can do about it.

Historically, humans ate food straight from the ground, fish from the ocean and rivers, and wild game or livestock when it was available. There weren't many degrees of separation between the two. There weren't fertilizers manufactured in factories or genetically modified seeds, just nature the way God made it. Our intestines worked well on a diet high in good fats, fiber, and nutrient dense foods.

Fast forward to today. Consider the rows and rows of pack-aged foods in the grocery store. Imagine the freezer cases and refrigeration cases full of food packaged to make your life easier. Now think about where the ingredients came from to make those items. How long ago was that corn harvested? What was the cow fed that provided the beef in that frozen shepherd's pie? What oil did they use to make this pastry? What is monosodium glutamate and hydrolyzed corn protein anyway? Why does this ice cream have 20 ingredients in it when all it needs to taste good is cream, sugar, and vanilla?

There are millions upon millions of dollars spent every year to catch your eye and money at the grocery store. The packag-ing, placement, and claims of these products look and sound too good to pass up. Ads pop up online, on Facebook, on TV, in magazines, on billboards, and on end caps at the market. We are consistently bombarded with marketing messages specifically designed to make us feel incomplete without the product being sold. Advertisers don't want you to realize you could live a happy life without what they are selling. It is their job to do all in their power to entice you to buy, buy, buy!

And as if their marketing messages weren't enough, food man-ufacturers add flavor enhancers and chemicals to our foods that increase appetite and food cravings. Even if one food company wants to produce only clean, simple foods for consumers they are bound by the fear of losing market share if their competitors' products are more appealing than theirs. If one company is using flavor enhancers and another is not, an uninformed public will simply buy the one that tastes better. The altruistic food producer then loses. It's similar to living in a time of scarcity where no one will share or do the right thing because they are afraid of being left with nothing. Fear is one of the Adversary's greatest tools. Fear is affecting our food supply and what we think of as food.

Where Does It Come From?

In his book *The Omnivore's Dilemma*, Michael Pollan follows the source ingredients from harvest to ingestion of four meals. Within the pages, many a light was shed on where the food we eat really comes from. I must warn you, it is not a pretty or appetizing story. Industrial feedlots, genetically modified corn, and factory-farmed eggs are not appealing places or things to begin with. But when you hear the detailed story of each you might start to get a little woozy.

I will abstain from recreating what Mr. Pollan managed to articulate so eloquently and spare you the wretched details. But I will tell you what it means for the human body. When food becomes a commodity to be bought and sold in faceless transactions, the integrity of its ability to nourish becomes questionable at best. **The farther your food travels from its harvest to your plate, the more nutrients are lost. The more food is altered and processed, the further the nutrients are depleted and the body has trouble recognizing it as food. The more pesticides and chemicals are added to food, the more dangerous it becomes for the human body.**

In the case of wheat, corn, and soy, hybridization and genetic modification has occurred by big business for several reasons:

1. To increase output
2. To raise resistance to pests
3. To make lots of money by patenting seed genetics and the pesticides that go with them

Notice none of these reasons include the intention to safely nourish and strengthen the health of those consuming the altered food. It all comes down to money and quarterly returns.

Food is big business. There are billions of dollars at stake. The only prayer individual consumers have of restoring the quality of food we eat is to forego the processing, boxing, and marketing and go straight to the source. We have to shop the outer edges of the grocery store; where the fresh items reside. We may have to skip grains for a while until someone is smart enough to plant and offer genetically un-modified varieties that have not been soaked in pesticides. But we have tremendous power individually and collectively to make positive changes by what we choose to buy.

Every time you spend money on food, you are casting a ballot. Every dollar sends a message. We don't need Congress to pass laws on our behalf telling us what we can and cannot eat. All we need is the freedom to choose and the transparency to know what is in the food we consume. Demand is a powerful predictor of supply. As women and mothers, we hold the lion's share of money spent on food. We must educate ourselves and our children on what is good for them and why. Food made from scratch, herbs grown on the windowsill, and knowing where your meat came from are good starting points. Farmers markets are popping up across America offering fresh ingredients straight from the source. Make a point to find one in your area and check out what it has to offer.

As a child of an overworked mother who was never taught how to cook herself, I have had to learn many things on my own. I wish that someone had shown me the way. In the book *Outliers, A Story of Success*, Malcolm Gladwell has a chapter on the 10,000 Hours to Success rule. He gathered data showing it takes around 10,000 hours of practice to become an expert at something. If children are taught early, they can invest those hours and become expert cooks and nutritionists before they start their own families. The alternative to being taught in your youth—attempting to learn how to cook as an adult while expected to simultaneously pay the bills and raise kids—is extremely difficult.

I lived on the worst food possible in college, graduated and got a good job in San Francisco. That job required a lot of travel. I survived on processed food, take-out, and restaurant food for years. At the same time my sister lived in Salt Lake City and traveled a different path. She worked in a fine-dining restaurant and became very knowledgeable about food sourcing and fresh ingredients. She would drag me to the farmers market downtown when I would fly in to visit for the weekend. In the mid to late 1990's I found it to be a little "earthy" for my tastes. In my snobbish mind (which was really just a front for being ignorant) I thought these people at the famers market must be desperate to shop that way. Couldn't they just go to the grocery store?

I was the one who would become desperate, as time would reveal.

What I have learned since then is that fresh food holds the energy and vitality of the earth. The longer we wait from harvest to consumption, the more that vitality is lost. There is a reason you can heal the body by going on a fresh, pesticide-free vegetable juice diet. It is because you supply the body with timely, intense nutrition and the enzymes it needs to tell those nutrients where to go. The earth was created perfectly and precisely to sustain life—that of plants, animals, and humans. It is no accident that the ecosystems found on the earth interact with each other in perfect balance. In that same way, specific plants and seeds are explicitly designed to sustain human life. Some may need soaking or fermenting before consumption, but they are intrinsically designed to support and nourish.

When mankind decided to hybridize and genetically alter our main food staples, I want to believe it was with the best of intentions. In the next chapter on wheat, we will cover a little of the history of this change. Those in power became gravely concerned about how to sustain an ever increasing human population. The result was a brain share symposium on how to solve the world's problems. I do not doubt the Adversary attended, whispering advice intended to create a more "well-fed" population. I am sure these ideas were delivered to men who were in a state of frantic worry and distress over the huge problem at hand. Were the decisions they finally made based on fear? Or were these decisions to alter the seeds mankind had been surviving on for millennia influenced by prayer and heavenly advice? We cannot know for sure. However, the changes that were first introduced have most certainly not been the last.

Agricultural businesses know they can patent genetically altered seeds and make big returns in two ways: first, by selling the "new and improved, pest resistant" seed, and second, by selling the pesticide that will kill everything but that seed. They design them to go together: the seed and the pesticide. It's a double win for the company's bottom line. The person who loses is the end consumer who ends up with an inflamed intestine because the foods they eat are no longer recognized as food. To underscore this point, check out www.geneticroulettemovie.com for more information on what genetically modified foods do to the human body.

Pesticides, preservatives, and other toxins also find their way into our food supply. I now try to avoid these things at all costs. If you do a little research on your own, you will find information on the chemicals put in and on our food. Watch the Yahoo clip titled, "Monsanto's Roundup® Herbicide—Featuring the Darth Vader Chemical," which explains new scientific discoveries on how this chemical, called glyphosate, could be causing cancer, gastrointestinal disorders, depression, infertility, heart disease, autism, diabetes, Alzheimer's, and obesity in America[11]. Additional detailed reasons to avoid pesticides and preservatives are found in the chapter titled Toxicity and Your Genetic Makeup. Here I will briefly summarize by saying the collective amount of toxins we ingest is beginning to overwhelm the human body—and that the more you purposefully avoid, the better off your gut and health will be.

Inflammation of your intestines is the beginning of food sensitivity and intolerance. I don't say "allergy" here because many doctors maintain a true allergy only occurs when there is a histamine reaction to a substance. Most people do not exhibit allergy-type symptoms to food intolerances. They exhibit other random symptoms like migraines, depression, muscle tension, back pain, arthritis, and attention deficit disorders. These random symptoms all come from inflammation and malnutrition.

When the gut becomes inflamed, it is because of an immune response to something we have knowingly or unknowingly ingested. Our bodies are designed to work this way. This high-alert response tells the gut's immunity army to sequester and disable any substance that has been deemed an invader. However, problems occur when the immune system gets either confused or overwhelmed. For example, say the gut has decided that wheat or soy is now an enemy to the body; you may be unknowingly introducing offensive substances multiple times a day, and the gut remains in a constant state of high-alert and inflammation. This causes poor absorption of nutrients and eventual malnourishment of the body's cells and tissues.

Our bodies are incredibly intelligent. If the intestine decides that it does not like a particular food, there is a reason for it. We may be low in enzymes to digest that food, or the food may often come paired with a noxious pesticide that we cannot break down. Another cause may be altered genetics within the food causing it to mimic a known enemy. The immune system within the gut operates on detection of cell exteriors. If a certain cell's shape has been registered as the enemy, anything mimicking that shape will also be attacked. It is the body's way of disallowing un-wanted particles to advance through the intestinal wall and into the bloodstream.

These layers of protection have served mankind well for thou-sands of years. It is just in the past fifty years or so that we have started to see rising cases of heart disease, diabetes, and obesity. Interestingly, in the past fifty years we have seen a rapid rise in ge-netically modified food consumption, although most people do not know it. Food manufacturers in the United States are current-ly not required to label whether a product contains genetically modified ingredients. There have been attempts in several states to change labeling laws to require full disclosure of genetically modified (also referred to as GMO) foods, but so far they have all been voted down. I wonder who might be behind the fight to keep the status quo; perhaps a force that wants mankind to be sick and miserable.

There are many documented cases of restored health by those who have eliminated genetically modified foods and embraced organic grains, meats, and produce[12]. Currently, common GMO foods in North America include soybeans, corn, canola, cotton-seed, and sugar from sugar beets.

The simple removal of toxic pesticides and genetically modi-fied food can calm the intestines and bring back health and vitality.

As a mother, I want to know exactly what I am feeding my children. And I know I am only one of many who feel the same. Since most food manufacturers are not including GMO informa-tion on their labels—I choose not to buy their products. Some food companies are thinking ahead; they do not use GMO ingre-dients and label their products willingly. As for the rest, I would suggest that your health and that of your family is not worth the convenience of these prepackaged foods. Check out www.

nongmoshoppingguide.com and the No GMO iTunes App for help in avoiding foods with GMOs.

As more and more consumers reject these foods a tipping point will occur. Demand will increase for non-GMO foods and farmers and food manufacturers will respond accordingly. Be part of the solution and choose your foods wisely. And if there are GMO labeling laws being put up for a vote in your state make sure you research the issue thoroughly and properly analyze the intent of heavily funded biotech infomercials. The health of your posterity could be at stake.

After years of exposure to altered and chemical-laden foods, you may find your intestines have developed sensitivities to specific things you eat. If you need to identify exact foods that may be causing your problems, the following section will tell you how.

How to Pinpoint Offending Foods Through Elimination, Lab Tests, or Rotation

If you suspect food intolerances are affecting your health, there are several methods to find the foods to which you react. The least expensive is a ***food elimination diet*** where you remove the foods you eat commonly for two weeks and then add them back to your diet one by one. The most common allergens are wheat, dairy, corn, soy, eggs, peanuts, tree nuts, and shellfish. But don't think that these are the only offenders. Vegetables, grains, chocolate, caffeine, sugar, artificial colors, and artificial sweeteners can also be triggers. Each food gets a two day reintroduction phase at the end of the two weeks whereby copious notes should be taken on how you feel. Reactions to a food can include headache, nausea, brain fog, anger, anxiety, or loss of concentration, among others. Any unwanted or undesirable feeling should be documented and considered.

Often, if you avoid an offending food for 90 days you can reset your body's immune response to it. But in other cases, such as with gluten, once an immune switch has been flipped it can be almost impossible to overcome. Be careful with food re-introduction and be prepared to avoid some foods for longer periods, if not permanently.

Another way to determine food sensitivities is with an *IgE, IgG food panel assessment* done in a lab. The IgE and IgG panels test for immune sensitivity within your body, not within your intestine. Blood is drawn and tested within a lab for blood antibody levels after exposure to certain foods. The body can have two response periods to an offending food: immediate-onset and delayed-onset hypersensitivity reactions. The IgE panel tests for immediate-onset hypersensitivity reactions and the IgG test looks for delayed reactions. These delayed reactions can occur up to 4 days after ingesting a food.

I was first tipped off about food sensitivities when going to an applied kinesiologist chiropractor. I was 31 years old and felt like I was 80. I also felt as if I was coming down with the flu every time I ate. He muscle tested me for a number of things (muscle testing is explained more fully in the chapter on Repatterning) and told me I had food intolerances. I did not believe him at first, questioning muscle testing entirely, but a blood test from US BioTek Laboratories showed me he was right. I have included sections of my results for you as an example. My immune system was fighting an all-out war every time I ate. If you have symptoms similar to these, your body may be doing the same. Notice on the charts at the left below the IgE results going off the chart? That is NOT normal, or desirable. The good news is that many of these sensitivities can be turned around. The charts on the right show my test results after 4 years of minimizing the offending foods and taking nutritional supplements:

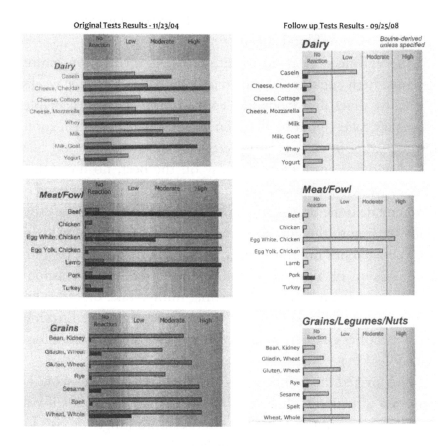

If your immune system goes into overdrive every time you eat, it is very likely that you have a leaky gut. Leaky gut syndrome occurs when the cells in the intestine walls become gapped and allow undigested foods to cross the intestinal barrier. Antibiotics, a lack of good bacteria, and wheat gluten can cause these gaps to occur.

To heal a leaky gut you need to take several steps. First, it is very likely your body has developed sensitivities to many of the foods you commonly eat. A leaky gut causes massive confusion among the protective forces of the immune system which starts to label once benign substances as problematic. This occurs because large molecules of the offending food are passing from the gut straight into your blood stream.

You will need to avoid wheat, dairy, eggs, corn, soy, grains, peanuts, high-sugar fruits, sugar, and chocolate for a few weeks. Eat easily digestible foods like cooked, non-starchy vegetables (squashes, sweet potato, all green veggies, parsnips), fish (non-farmed salmon, cod, herring, etc.), organic chicken and beef raised without antibiotics (go easy on the beef, no more than once a week), and no more than a handful of nuts per day. Homemade bone broths as a base for soups and sauces are especially healing to the gut. Start the day with a smoothie made of unsweetened nut milk, some berries, greens, brown rice protein, a tablespoon of almond or sunflower butter, and a teaspoon of L-Glutamine to heal the intestinal lining. Take digestive enzymes with each meal (covered in more depth in the Enzymes and Probiotics chapter) to assist with proper breakdown of food molecules.

I discovered this protocol through trial and error and with the help of a nutritionist. It helped my body immensely. But if you are skeptical, read *Clean Gut* by Dr. Alejandro Junger or visit his website at www.cleangut.com. His book helped connect the final dots on why this protocol worked. He explains how the layers of the gut interact, how they become imbalanced, and which natural supplements help restore optimal function. His work is based on decades of experience as a certified M.D., healing others, and trying to find his own path back to health.

Once your several weeks of clean eating are over, carefully reintroduce common dietary foods. You will find that after weeks of eating in a new way, you don't have a desire for sugar or pastries. You may desire to stay on that path and enjoy former offending foods only occasionally. Either way, pay attention to how these foods make you feel and omit them accordingly. Be warned that reduced cravings and a clearer mind may lead you to choose this new way of eating for life.

Another way to heal from food sensitivities is a ***rotation diet***. A rotation diet requires that you not eat a food more than one day out of four. For example, you could eat beef and rice on Mondays, chicken and corn on Tuesdays, fish and wheat on Wednesdays, and turkey and quinoa on Thursdays and then start the rotation over again. Obviously this is extremely simplified as you would be eating other items as well, but the trick is to not eat a food for more than 24 hours in any 96 hour period. Scientists have discovered it takes approximately 96 hours for all traces of a food to completely exit your system. This allows the immune system to "flame down" between exposures and maintain a lower level of reaction. You may take your 24 hour periods from dinner one day to mid-day the next so you can eat leftovers from the night before for lunch.

However you may choose to uncover and pinpoint if you have food sensitivities, do not be scared of the findings. There are many books and blogs that cover allergen-free eating. Making the change nowadays is much easier than it was ten years ago. And the freedom from all the effects of food sensitivities can be life-altering in many positive ways.

Unfortunately, there are two specific foods in our diets that are starting to cause an increasing amount of trouble. They are so pervasive in our culture that each one deserves a closer look. The next two chapters cover the origins and modifications of our two most beloved foods: wheat and dairy.

Chapter 6

WHEAT FOR MAN?

How and Why Our Favorite Food Is Making Us Sick

My personal love affair with wheat began around the age of eight. I suddenly could not get enough bread, bagels, pie crusts, biscuits, fried fruit pies, doughnuts, pizza, sandwiches, croutons, rolls, buns, and cookies. If it had wheat in it, I was all over it. Not coincidentally, I'm sure, I started gaining weight around that time. I went from a normal eight year-old girl to a roly-poly young woman. I was painfully aware that I no longer looked like my healthy-sized friends, but at that time I didn't know how to lose weight. I certainly didn't have the will power to simply cut calories. All I knew was that eating anything made with wheat flour made me incredibly happy.

I struggled with weight loss for the next 30 years. I went to diet centers, exercised excessively, tried self-control (which always failed miserably), and followed plans in magazines. If I ever lost weight, it always found me again. One time after being on an extremely strict diet for six weeks, I remember giving in and eating a toasted bagel with butter. It tasted like heaven itself. The tears rolled down my cheeks as I realized I was completely powerless against food.

From all my experiments in weight loss, however, I did start to notice a pattern. It didn't matter what diet I was on, if it didn't completely cut out wheat and sugar, I would not lose weight. I couldn't have just "a little" bread and stick to a diet. After eating anything with wheat, I would begin to crave it so badly my resolve completely disappeared. And forget anything with flour AND sugar—I was helpless to the power of that combination unless it was avoided completely. I simply could not lose weight without eliminating those two things. And those two things were the absolute hardest things to give up.

Flash forward to 2004. I had seen several different kinds of doctors to try and figure out my nebulous health problems: fatigue, trouble sleeping, feeling "tired but wired," circles under my eyes, hair that stopped growing, brain fog, constant sadness, getting flu-like symptoms every time I ate, inability to feel joy, and no connection to God. One doctor ran a blood test for food allergies and discovered my immune system was reacting to almost everything I ate on a regular basis. The test also showed I was intolerant to wheat. I then went to a hormone clinic and was diagnosed with Hashimoto's thyroiditis. Hashimoto's is an autoimmune disease which occurs when your body starts fighting against your own thyroid tissue.

At that point, I didn't understand any of the interconnectivity of my symptoms. That slowly unfolded over the next nine years as I fought, studied, and stumbled my way through some horrible times. I hope and pray you will not experience what I did—so in this chapter you will learn what you need to know to regain or protect the health of yourself and those you love.

We will cover a history of wheat, issues from wheat consumption, and signs you should look for to determine if wheat is a problem for you. You will also learn how long you need to avoid wheat to determine a true sensitivity.

The History of Wheat

Thousands of years ago, humans ate a pure, ancient version of wheat called einkorn wheat. Einkorn wheat has 14 chromosomes. This is important to know because wheat has the genetic ability to add upon its own genetic structure when cross-bred or exposed to the pollen of another viable grass or grain. A later version of einkorn wheat is emmer wheat, which cross-bred with goat grass and retained 28 chromosomes (14 from einkorn and 14 from the goat-grass). Later still, emmer wheat naturally cross-bred with another grass and gained 14 more chromosomes. Stabilizing at 42-chromosomes, this version of wheat is the closest to that which was eaten for thousands of years by our ancestors.

Anciently people ate it as a soaked porridge and later learned how to make flatbreads. Later still, the people learned how to leaven the wheat and make bread loaves. As our ancestors traveled from land to land and across the seas, they brought wheat with them to plant, cultivate, and feed their offspring. As recently as the 1950's, this 42-chromosomal wheat was the same stuff growing and feeding Americans, Europeans, Indians, and other cultures around the world.

In the mid-1940's, and as a result of World War II, there was great concern on how to feed the world's growing population. Many were starving or malnourished because of the effects of the war. From a noble effort to stamp out world hunger, geneticist Dr. Norman Borlaug developed exceptionally high-yielding dwarf wheat using cytogenic hybridization. This wheat is credited with increasing crop output eight-fold. In 1970, Dr. Borlaug won the Congressional Gold Medal and the Nobel Peace Prize for his efforts. His hybridized version of wheat filtered through most of the United States and much of the rest of the world.

The problem with this hybridized wheat is that there were zero clinical trials or lab-tests to check for effects on human consumption. Scientists assumed that since the final product was still wheat-like, that changes in gluten content and cell structure would be harmless. And since the problem of global hunger was so pervasive, out went any thoughts of possible damage to humans. The new wheat strain entered our fields and markets without ceremony or protest. The question is—has this new (and altered again in the 1990's) strain of wheat had any negative effects on the human population?

Issues with Wheat Consumption

The following list contains known complications from wheat ingestion. However, it is not exhaustive:

- **Wheat polypeptides have the peculiar ability to penetrate the blood-brain barrier and bind to the brain's morphine receptors** (the same receptor to which opiate drugs bind) **to create a mild euphoria.**
- **Wheat can exacerbate symptoms of schizophrenia[13].**
- **Wheat is a known appetite stimulant.** Because it can also block appetite satiation receptors, causing one to overeat even when full, it is a favorite ingredient of food manufacturers who want increased consumption of their products[14].
- **Wheat causes visceral fat accumulation in the abdomen.** This type of fat is located around the visceral organs: the liver, kidneys, pancreas, intestines, and belly. It is unique in that it has the ability to produce inflammatory signals

and abnormal cell communication hormones. These confusing signals sent out to the rest of the body wreak havoc on the endocrine system. **Visceral fat is connected to the cause of diabetes, dementia, rheumatoid arthritis, and colon cancer[15] [16].** Visceral fat also creates surplus estrogen which adds to the risk of breast cancer in women and growth of breast tissue in men.

- **The hybridized wheat we eat today increases blood sugar more quickly and to a higher degree than table sugar[17].** The glycemic index is a number between 1 and 100 that indicates a food's impact on the body's blood sugar levels, and is commonly referred to as the "GI" number. The GI for whole wheat bread is 72. White sugar has a glycemic index of 59. [Please note: the only foods higher than whole wheat bread on the GI scale are corn starch, rice starch, potato starch, and tapioca starch. BEWARE— these are the same ingredients many manufacturers put into gluten-free processed foods. Stay away from ingredients with a high GI!] Because of wheat's ability to raise blood sugar so quickly, it also causes a higher spike in insulin in the body. More insulin means more visceral fat deposits, and a never-ending cycle of cravings and blood sugar dips and spikes.

- **Wheat consumption triggers Celiac disease.** Celiac disease is a disorder that occurs when eating gluten causes damage to the lining of the small intestines. The disease does not usually manifest itself initially with intestinal discomfort. It often begins with nebulous signals such as fatigue or migraines. It takes an average of 11 years for most people with Celiac disease to be diagnosed. Sufferers usually develop a severely malnourished state (especially low in B vitamins) because the cilia in their intestines, small hair-like receptors in the gut responsible for nutrient delivery, lay flat and damaged instead of upright and functioning. **Celiac disease has increased four hundred percent in the past 50 years**[18].

- **Eliminating wheat from the diet results in 350-400 less calories consumed per day on average with no other dietary changes required.** It has also been proven to decrease cravings and appetite.

- **Forty percent of the population has one or more antibody markers that predispose them to Celiac disease, yet show no apparent symptoms.**

- **Wheat gliadin (a protein in wheat gluten) has recently been proven to trigger the intestines to release a protein called zonulin. Zonulin dissolves the tough bindings between intestinal cell walls that protect the gut from allowing unwanted substances from the intestines into the blood stream**[19]. Also called "leaky gut syndrome," this leakage of proteins into the bloodstream causes a myriad of inflammatory conditions such as celiac, asthma, and joint issues.

- **Wheat gluten is so similar to thyroid tissue that if gluten enters the blood stream through a leaky gut, the internal immune system can become confused.** It sometimes attacks both the foreign gluten proteins and its own thyroid tissue, resulting in thyroid disease.

- **Unresolved celiac disease can result in the following seemingly unrelated conditions: malnutrition, liver disease, autoimmune issues, neurological impairment, insulin-dependent diabetes, and dermatitis.**

- **Finally, wheat crops have been increasingly sprayed with glyphosate, the key ingredient in Roundup®** [20]. **This chemical has been shown to cause disruptions in**

gut bacteria, leaky gut, depletion of vital minerals, vitamins, and nutrients, and impair cytochrome enzymes that aid the liver in detoxifying environmental toxins[21].

Battling Wheat: A True Story

For some people, wheat is an addictive substance. I learned firsthand that the connection between wheat consumption and brain chemistry is real. Wheat can be so addictive to some that it can seem impossible to give up.

It took five years from the time I was told I was intolerant to wheat to the point I had enough internal strength to attempt a long-term separation. To me, it seemed that everything delicious had wheat in it—absolutely everything. I couldn't mentally handle the thought of a life devoid of pizza, sandwiches, rolls, and cookies. I would try a few days of separation and felt absolutely terrible. Logically I decided that the doctor's test must have been wrong and that eliminating gluten wasn't the answer to my random, seemingly unconnected health issues. Then I would end my ban on gluten (very happily, I might add) and enjoy all the things I should have been avoiding. I would feel a euphoric rush and just *knew* that gluten was not a problem for me. Eating it made me feel great, and eliminating it made me feel terrible. How could avoiding it be a good thing for me?

On the other hand, I felt awful most of the rest of the time. I had brain fog that became so bad I often felt as if I were in a stupor. Remembering things was incredibly difficult. I lived in fear that my impaired memory and brain function would be discovered by my employers or people I volunteered with at church and my children's school. I was very sensitive to loud noises and chaos—I had to escape it. I could not exercise at my gym because they had eight TVs playing different stations and music piped through the entire exercise floor. The amount of information overload was more than my brain could handle. Too much sound and light made me feel angry and anxious. My poor kids had to hear me say constantly: "Please speak more quietly. I am right next to you!"

In addition, I was very vulnerable to the criticisms of others. I tried my very best to avoid making mistakes or causing a scene that would draw attention to me. I was like a scared, hunched-over woman just trying to get through the day. I also became paranoid that people didn't like me. If someone failed to respond to a text or call, I immediately assumed they didn't want to interact with me. If an aquaintance didn't smile or say hi as I walked by I took it personally and began to analyze what I did wrong. I filed every possible slight internally and kept it all to myself. I kept all potential friends at arm's length because I couldn't handle the possibility of being rejected or not included. It was much easier to play defense than put myself out there and get hurt.

Long ago, when I was a four year-old attending preschool, I remember a particular day very clearly. Two of the preschool teachers asked me if I would see-saw with a new student. The new student was deaf and very sensitive to facial expressions, the teachers explained. They asked if I would smile and encourage her as we see-sawed so she would feel comfortable. I said I would and we started our up and down playing. I smiled and she smiled back happily. Then I began to wonder: what would happen if I frowned at her? Being just four years of age and very curious, I made a bad choice. As the teachers looked away, I made a mad face just to see what would happen. She immediately started screaming and crying and begged to get off the see-saw. I was devastated that what I had done had made her so unhappy. I felt terrible. To this day, I have never forgotten that event.

The sad irony is that I got to know exactly how she felt that day later in my life. My own paranoia of being disliked intensified through my thirties. It was constant and debilitating. I made no close friends for almost a decade and felt incredibly lonely. I tried my very best to fly under the radar and go unseen because I couldn't "read" others or make good friendships. I highly doubt anyone knew of my problem because I became very good at faking normal behavior. I probably just appeared snobby or aloof. Heaven forbid someone should discover my weakness—a sad commentary on my state of mind.

Life also didn't seem worth living. There was no joy. I had two healthy children and a wonderful, loving husband and I still could not feel joy. It just wasn't there. Even on anti-depressants, the wonder at why anyone would want to live a long life resonated with me. I would pray that Heavenly Father wouldn't make me live on the earth longer than absolutely necessary. I pleaded not to have to live past 75. That age seemed plenty long to me—and far longer than I wanted on most days.

To put these things in perspective, none of these symptoms existed until after I had a difficult ovarian surgery, massive work stress, and two extremely difficult pregnancies. It was as if I had strained my body past a certain threshold, a switch had been thrown, and I could not seem to regain my former health. But there is a light at the end of this tunnel.

When I finally removed wheat from my diet for an extended period of time, almost all of these symptoms disappeared. The depression lifted. The paranoia evaporated. The sensitivity to light and sound was gone. And best of all, I began to be able to feel joy again. My desire to go to church resurfaced. I actually wanted to reconnect with God.

It did not solve every health problem, but it did correct many.

These days if I consume wheat, I immediately feel a heightened sense of sound and irritability. For the next 24 hours, life becomes dark and overwhelming. I have a hard time remembering things and the brain fog returns. The signs are much easier to interpret now that I have been gluten-free for a long period of time. When I was eating gluten regularly, the signs were more convoluted and harder to pinpoint to a cause. If I avoided wheat for only a few days the symptoms did not go away and the withdrawal symptoms were severe. So in the short term, I thought there was no connection to my health problems because it definitely didn't make me feel better. It took an extended period of being gluten-free to connect the symptoms with the actual cause.

If you experience depression, migraines, heightened sensitivity to light or sound, paranoia, anxiety, or severe insecurity **it is very likely you have a gluten sensitivity.** It is worth your time and effort to eliminate it from your diet for 90 days. Your body needs at least three months (at minimum!) to heal from extensive gut damage from a lifetime of eating wheat. Some experts say to avoid a possible offending food for two weeks. Then re-introduce the food and watch for negative reactions. I know that my addiction to wheat could not be detoxed in two weeks. I suggest 90 days of super-clean gluten-free living to get the truest results.

I also strongly recommend taking a teaspoon of powdered L-glutamine in water up to three times a day. L-glutamine nourishes your intestinal cilia and can help heal damage from years of abuse. Once your cilia re-awaken, your ability to absorb nutrients and heal the rest of the body will increase significantly.

You may have noticed that the symptoms I described above are the same as those of many autistic children. Wheat has been shown to exacerbate common symptoms of autism: sensitivity to light and sound, social anxiety, and brain fog. I have several friends whose autistic children became very highly functioning once they remove wheat from their diets. This is also something to consider if you have a child who suffers from social anxiety or learning disorders. All these symptoms are related and they most likely start in the gut. Once you remove gut offenders and heal the intestinal lining, a whole new world could emerge for your child.

The Word of Wisdom

In The Church of Jesus Christ of Latter-day Saints we follow a health protocol called The Word of Wisdom. In Doctrine and Covenants Section 89 verses 16-17 it states, "All grain is good for the food of man; as also the fruit of the vine; that which yieldeth fruit, whether in the ground or above the ground—Nevertheless, **wheat for man**, and corn for the ox, and oats for the horse, and rye for the fowls and for swine, and for all beasts of the field, and barley for all useful animals, and for mild drinks, as also other grain."

When I was told I shouldn't eat wheat, the Word of Wisdom phrase "wheat for man" immediately entered my mind. It swirled and danced in my head for years causing me to question the Word of Wisdom and its source. I felt broken and out of place in a community where everyone else was storing bags of red winter wheat for food storage and grinding it to make their own bread. Why was I the odd one out?

I finally began to analyze my physical history and realized I had endured huge amounts of mental and physical stress for extended periods of time. I had not managed the stress, or attempted to get out from under it. I didn't know about meditation or stress-reducing breathing exercises or how dangerous extensive stress could be. I had simply hung on and endured. But by simply enduring without supporting my health, my body had paid a high price. I hadn't been eating properly or taking vitamins to give the body assistance during the hard times. I didn't realize that stress can break the immune system into malfunction. As a result, my body had been pushed past a point of no return. My hope is that you can avoid this same fate by increasing your nutrient intake and using some of the techniques found later in the chapter on stress.

If you suffer from gluten intolerance or celiac disease, it is not a stamp of inferiority from God. It is a shortcoming in the body that is triggered by hybridized modifications to wheat, leaky intestinal walls, and nutrient-poor diets. Starting in the gut, wheat intolerance causes severe reactions which manifest themselves in random ways. In addition, wheat continues to be experimented upon and altered by scientists and corporations. All these facts create a recipe for health disaster.

Another point to consider is this: from reading the Bible, we learn that Jesus broke bread with his disciples to institute the first sacrament. In my church and many others, we continue this practice to this day. The bread signifies the body of Christ, which was shed for us. When we partake of it, we are to remember Him and the great sacrifice that was made. On the opposing side, the Adversary hates when we listen to Christ. He twists and changes the truth to confuse and ensnare the children of God every day. Has the Adversary urged man to alter the very substance of the symbol of Christ's gift—the bread—at its source? The very structure that nourishes the wheat berries resulting in gluten content has been unarguably altered. Just like changes to ancient texts of scripture that confuse the mind of man, perhaps the genetic changes to wheat have been created to confuse the body of man. While many people may not partake of the knowledge held within the scriptures, almost every single person eats wheat in his or her lifetime. If Satan cannot get you to avoid or turn away from God's truth, perhaps he has devised a second way to keep you from God: physical depression, illness, confusion, and misery.

I finally reconciled wheat intolerance and the advice held in the Word of Wisdom. The wheat we eat today is not the same substance it was 100 years ago. It has been altered by mankind in many ways. I have no doubt the Adversary has had a hand in the modification of wheat. Think of the amount of pain and suffering caused among the overweight, diabetic, arthritic, and those with celiac disease. Then think about the pain passed along to their spouses, children, extended family, and friends.

I also have a second theory about the cause of wheat intolerance. I would not be surprised if unwanted bacteria, viruses, and/or fungi find their way into our digestive system and either feed on the modified wheat, or find little resistance to their invasion because of a confused immune system from wheat hybridizations and pesticides applied to the crops. Having personally endured years of food allergies changing and morphing, I know wheat consumption can cause ever-changing immune issues in a person with a weakened constitution. When I avoid wheat, my body's immune system seems to quit "fighting at nothing" and draining precious energy reserves.

For the record, I never had intestinal pain or any kind of digestive distress signals during these times. If you think only people with intestinal issues may have gluten intolerance, you are mistaken. You may be suffering needlessly because you are experiencing no symptoms at the source. Please consider this as you ascertain whether or not gluten could be causing your health problems. Give yourself a break from gluten and see if your symptoms resolve. It may take many weeks to notice positive changes start to occur, but it is well worth the sacrifice.

To guide you in this process, check out gluten-free cookbooks and blogs (one of my favorites is www.glutenfreegirl.com). There are more and more products and restaurant options for those sensitive to gluten. Do note that gluten is found in more foods than you may realize: salad dressings, monosodium glutamate, "natural flavors," soy sauce, and other convenience foods are riddled with it. As mentioned previously, try not to replace wheat with large amounts of gluten-free packaged foods and baked goods as they are usually made with potato or tapioca starches that cause rapid spikes in blood sugar. If you are suffering from hormonal issues and/or depression, blood sugar instability may be one of the causes and you would only be trading one problem for another. A better bet is to try some of the Paleo cookbooks that use coconut, almond, and arrowroot flours and are designed to have a low glycemic index (a smaller effect on your blood sugar levels). I found this to be one of the confusing issues I discovered after abstaining from wheat which caused me to question the initial results. If you also encounter conflicting results, make sure to read the chapter on candida—it may be another issue you need to consider.

Now that you know more about wheat, let's discuss our next favorite food source: dairy.

Chapter 7
MILK DOES A BODY…
The Truth about Dairy

I grew up with milk as a constant companion. In my family we had milk every morning at breakfast, milk with lunch at school, milk and cookies after school, and sometimes ice cream after dinner. We also ate plenty of yogurt and cheese. All of it was delicious!

There are numerous advertisements about how good milk is for the body and how important it is for proper growth in children. It has calcium, protein, vitamin D (added), and other nutrients. How could it be anything but good for us?

During my health journey, I was shocked when a doctor informed me I was very sensitive to dairy. I didn't want to eliminate dairy products from my diet. I love milk and all products that are made from it, but I couldn't ignore the fact that I felt awful after eating or drinking them. I just didn't understand how milk could be the cause. So I rolled up my sleeves, did some research, and realized more people should be aware of the truth about dairy.

In this chapter you will learn the history of milk and why some ethnic groups are more suited to its consumption than others. You will also learn what affects the quality of the milk you drink: from what cows are fed, to pasteurization and homogenization. All these factors should be considered as you choose your milk sources or whether to consume dairy at all.

Milk and Our Ancestors

The discovery of milk fat particulates on ancient pottery shards as old as 6000 B.C. have led to the belief that the people of Great Britain and Northern Europe were among the first to use cows' milk for human consumption. Scientists believe that a genetic mutation called lactase-persistence (which allowed milk consumption and lactose digestion after a child was weaned and onwards into adulthood) appeared between 5000-4000 B.C. The Sumerians were proven to have started using dairy around 3000 B.C. from ancient carvings and pottery work that showed the people straining milk to make butter and cheese. The ancient Egyptians and Indians domesticated and/or worshipped cows starting in 3000 B.C. and 2000 B.C. respectively. The ancient Hebrews used milk abundantly as evidenced in ancient texts. The Bible itself has around fifty references to milk and milk products.

In essence, the human population (depending on region) has had a long relationship with milk. Asian and African populations seem to have the shortest history or exposure to milk. As you can see in the table below, it seems that lactose intolerance is highly related to how long the people of a region have used milk as part of their diets.

Lactose Intolerance by Ethnicity

Ethnicity	Percent Lactose Intolerant	Ethnicity	Percent Lactose Intolerant
British (U.K.)	5-15%[1]	Balkans Region	55%[1]
German (Germany)	15%[1]	Jewish (North America)	60-80%[3]
Austrian (Austria)	15-20%[1]	French (Southern France)	65%[1]
Finnish (Finland)	17%[1]	Indian (Southern India)	70%[1]
French (Northern France)	17%[1]	African (Africa)	70-90%[1]
Italian (Italy)	20-70%[1]	African American (North America)	75%[2]
Anglo (North America)	21%[2]	Central Asian	80%[1]
Indian (Northern India)	30%[1]	Native American (North America)	80-100%[3]
Hispanic (North America)	51%[2]	East Asian	90-100%[1]

Sources:
1. Michael de Vrese, MD "Probiotics: Compensation for Lactase Insufficiency," *American Journal of Clinical Nutrition,* Feb., 2001
2. Nevin S. Scrimshaw, MD "The Acceptability of Milk and Milk Products in Populations with a High Prevalence of Lactose Intolerance," *American Journal of Clinical Nutrition,* Oct., 1988
3. National Institute of Child Health and Human Development "Lactose Intolerance: Information for Health Care Providers," NIH Publication No. 05-5303B, Jan., 2006

Descendants of Britain and Northern Europe are the most well-equipped to tolerate dairy and dairy products. Asians and those of African descent should probably avoid dairy like the plague.

The human body is made to tolerate mother's milk until sometime between the ages of four to six. After six years of age, milk may no longer be tolerable for many people. According to an article in BMC Evolutionary Biology, "An estimated 65% of human adults (and most adult mammals) downregulate [decrease] the production of intestinal lactase after weaning. Lactase is necessary for the digestion of lactose, the main carbohydrate in milk, and without it, milk consumption can lead to bloating, flatulence, cramps and nausea. Continued production of lactase throughout adult life (lactase persistence, LP) is a genetically determined trait and is found at moderate to high frequencies in Europeans and some African, Middle Eastern and Southern Asian populations.[22]"

Unfortunately, most of us don't know these facts and just eat what everyone else around us is eating. If you live in the United States, you probably eat dairy every day. It is a large part of our diet. Unfortunately, you may not have been granted the magic milk gene that allows you to consume dairy at such frequent intervals—if at all. Consider your ancestry and re-consider your consumption of dairy. You may become a much happier person without it.

More Recently

Two hundred years ago, if you wanted some milk, you most likely would have milked the family cow or bought milk from a neighbor with a cow. The fat in the milk would have floated to the top and been partially skimmed off to make butter and buttermilk. The rest of the milk would be drunk by the glass, after being shaken to incorporate the remaining fat, or used in recipes for the enjoyment of all.

Today, if you have ever tasted raw, unpasteurized milk, you are among an elite minority. Unless you grew up on or near a farm that had milking cows, your access to raw milk has greatly diminished thanks to some whisky distilleries in New York in the late 19th century. The story of what actually occurred follows.

Starting around the mid-1800's, typhoid and tuberculosis began spreading like wildfire in and around New York. The outbreak especially affected babies and young children and caused a rapid increase in infant mortality. The local officials finally determined the source of the outbreak to be the milk coming out of several nearby distillery farms. These distilleries used grains to produce their whiskey and other alcohols. The by-product of the distilleries was known as swill (spent grains). The distilleries' dilemma was what to do with all the swill after the alcohol was produced. It was decided that they would open dairy farms, feed it to cows, and make profit from the refuse.

Unfortunately, the swill was so stripped of nutrients that the milk these cows provided was bluish in color and contained such poor fats that they couldn't even be used for butter or cheese. These distillery farms had reportedly unsanitary conditions for their cows as well. Because of these circumstances, the milk taken from these cows was contaminated. It was then sold to the public with typhoid, tuberculosis, and many lives lost as the result.

Enter Louis Pasteur, the French chemist and biologist. Through his life's work, he endeavored to prove that food-borne illnesses and infectious diseases were caused by "germs." The creator of "Germ Theory," Pasteur went on to show that harmful microbes in milk caused sickness in humans. He then discovered that rapidly heating then cooling the milk killed most of these germs. Pasteurization was born. In 1895, commercial pasteurization machines were introduced in the United States.

Pasteurization has no doubt saved countless lives over the last century. Food processors are required by law to pasteurize milk and juices for the safety of the larger population. And when large, faceless manufacturing plants are turning out our food, it makes perfect sense. Unfortunately, when milk is pasteurized the enzyme lactase, along with many other enzymes which occur naturally in milk, is destroyed. Lactase is required to break-down lactose, the sugar found in milk. Those with lactose intolerance know all too well that consuming dairy without any lactase support can be extremely painful—including gas, bloating, and diarrhea. And lactase is just one example. Pasteurization kills all enzymes. There is an entire chapter on enzymes coming up that you must read to understand why this is such a travesty. To put it mildly, in today's modern world we need all the enzymes we can get.

Another issue with our current milk supply is homogenization. Homogenization is the process whereby large fat globules in milk are broken down into tiny fat globules. This keeps the fat from separating to the top. It is apparently a necessary convenience for milk drinkers everywhere to not have to shake their milk containers each day to incorporate the fat. But there's just one tiny little problem with homogenization: the fat particles become so small they can cross a compromised intestinal barrier and head straight into your bloodstream without being digested. After these particles enter your bloodstream, they are interpreted as an "enemy" because of their undigested, unrecognizable form. The high alert is sounded and the fight ensues. The immune system does its very best to disarm this invader but doesn't quite know how to win the fight. This whole process causes chaos in the immune system. The result is hypersensitivity to your environment, along with food and outdoor allergies.

A third problem with milk today is artificial growth bovine hormones. Known as rBST, or rBgh, this substance increases milk production in cows and is a genetically engineered growth hormone. It was approved for commercial use by the FDA on November 5, 1993. An FDA advisory committee concluded that "the use of rBST—and any increased risk of mastitis and resulting increased use of antibiotics in treated cattle—would not pose a risk to human health[23]." Logic would disagree. When you inject hormones into an animal that cause mastitis which leads to antibiotic use, and then drink the milk of that animal, you may very likely be affected by both the antibiotics and the hormones.

Finally, cows fed pesticide-laden, genetically modified corn could pull those chemicals into the milk they produce. The very nature of the chemical glyphosate in pesticides kills weeds and pests by blocking vitamin and mineral absorption (or by causing inflammation and eruption of the intestines of pests). This could result in reduced nutrient content from the modified corn that is engineered to handle large amounts of pesticides. The next logical step would mean fewer nutrients in the milk produced as well as an increase in chemical compounds.

Cows' stomachs are designed to eat grasses. When they are fed corn, gastrointestinal distress is the result. When they are fed genetically modified corn, the effects are even worse[24]. What cows are fed affects their milk production and the quality of the meat they produce. You are what you eat.

Effects of Dairy

When I was a teenager, I longed for beautiful skin. I looked at others and wondered why their skin was so perfect and mine so imperfect. In Austin, Texas, as of 2013, there is a billboard by a local high school that says "Milk causes acne in teens"—and its message is correct. Milk has now been shown to cause and exacerbate acne[25]. For some teens, monthly acne outbreaks are often hormone related, and can subside when food sources containing additional hormones are removed from the diet. Because of the nature of hormonal changes during the teen years, the last thing teenagers need is hormones in the foods they eat.

This is evidenced by the fact that girls are reaching puberty earlier than ever. Researchers cite diets high in meat and milk products as the cause. By starting their menstrual cycles earlier, our daughters have more hormones throughout their lives and an increased risk of type-2 diabetes later on in life[26]. This puts them at a higher risk for breast, ovarian, and uterine cancers.

Milk is also connected to rheumatoid arthritis and other joint problems[27]. Numerous studies correlate dairy consumption to joint issues. If you have pain in your joints, avoid milk and dairy for a time. See how you feel and adjust your diet accordingly.

According to www.austismspeaks.org, the current odds of an American child being diagnosed with autism are 1 in 68. Dairy can be highly inflammatory to some children's digestive systems. This can exacerbate the symptoms of autism or result in autism-like indicators. I have one friend whose young son was showing definitive signs of autism. On a whim she decided to change their family's milk supply to a raw, organic source. All of his autism markers disappeared. I have another friend who took her non-speaking autistic son off of dairy and wheat, and watched him begin to speak for the first time.

Finally, milk triggers mucus production. In the intestinal tract, this hampers digestion and absorption of vitamins. In the sinuses, this can lead to inflammation, sinus infections and over-use of antibiotics. Antibiotic over-use is causing more problems than we realize. More details on this topic will be found in the chapter on enzymes and probiotics.

In Summary

Milk today isn't what it was 200 years ago. Pasteurization, homogenization, and altered livestock diets all affect what ends up in your fridge. Milk consumption has been connected to allergies, acne, arthritis, and early adolescence in girls. You may want to consider eliminating commercially processed milk from you and your family's diet.

If you can tolerate dairy, raw (unpasteurized, un-homogenized) milk—when taken from healthy, grass-fed cows under sanitary conditions—is the ultimate form of milk. See www.raw-milk-facts.com for more information. If you have access to raw milk—go for it! And happily consume butter and cheese from these cows.

If you consume dairy and don't have access to this kind of milk (which is most likely the case, since as of this writing 17 states have deemed it illegal, and all other states have strict raw-milk sales laws), make sure it is organic. Avoid commercially-processed dairy from cows fed GMO corn and injected with rBST. And if you avoid milk entirely, take a calcium and vitamin D supplement in addition to your daily multi-vitamins. Your body will thank you.

Chapter 8
ENZYMES AND PROBIOTICS:
The Secret Powerhouses of the Human Body

Just outside our widow there are magical things happening every day. Grass grows, flowers bloom, and the animals go about their business. Water flows down rivers and into lakes and then into the ocean. Bumblebees flaunt their lack of concern for physics and fly about anyway, pollinating the flowers as they go. Squirrels play and gardens grow. In the fall, the shadows lengthen, plants go dormant, and in the spring, the cycle of life begins all over again.

When plants or trees die, they magically become earth again through a process of biodegradation. There are bugs that eat wood or plant matter and turn it back into soil. Molds and fungi break down dead things and feed others as they go. If an animal dies, its body decomposes back into the earth. Microorganisms break down both plant and flesh, and the earth then uses the nutrients from the whole process to feed new life. In its entirety, it is an amazing, self-perpetuating cycle that doesn't require any input from humankind. Nature just does its thing, year after year.

Our bodies are similar to nature in many ways. Cells are created, work hard and then die. Other processes clean up the dead cells and break them down or carry them away. Food is eaten, broken down to be used for fuel, and then carried out as waste. We don't have to think about any of these processes—they just happen. In fact, the more our brains stay out of the way, the happier our bodies are.

We've already talked about how the gut is the second brain and how the brain is affected by what happens in the intestines. But where does the entire digestion process really start? Or rather, where is the first place problems can occur to cascade down to the rest of the system? The answer is: within the body's enzyme production system.

What are Enzymes?

Enzymes are proteins that are chemical catalysts to digestion and many other processes within the body. There are both digestive enzymes and metabolic enzymes produced internally. These substances are the spark that starts a desirable chemical "flame," or process inside the body. Enzymes begin the processes of digestion and energy conversion when food is consumed. Sometimes an enzyme needs an additional component to do its job properly, called a coenzyme. Common coenzymes are magnesium, zinc, and potassium. Vitamins are necessary to produce some coenzymes that assist in the production of energy within our body. Enzymes are usually required to complete a cycle of chemical processes—without them at each proper step, the cycle cannot be completed.

To illustrate, once you begin thinking about eating, your

mouth begins to salivate. This saliva contains amylase that breaks down carbohydrates into their component sugars while you chew. Once the food arrives in your stomach, acid and protease enzymes (called pepsin) released by the stomach spend about 60 minutes breaking down the food further so that nutrients from the food can be absorbed in the small intestine. Once in the small intestine, additional enzymes are released to break down sugars, starches, and proteins so they can be absorbed and used for energy by all the cells in the body.

Since we now understand the connection between the gut and our brains, let's explore what could possibly go wrong with the digestive system.

Possible Problems in the Intestines

- Lack of vitamins or minerals to produce coenzymes
- Poor chewing to start the digestive process
- Lack of stomach acid (common as we age) to properly break down food before entering the small intestine
- Lack of pepsin in the stomach
- Inflammation in the intestines from yeast, food sensitivities, toxins, or parasites which inhibits enzyme production and thus, proper breakdown of food particles
- All the above leading to a "leaky gut" that allows food to cross the intestinal barrier before it is fully digested, which puts the white blood cells of our immune system on high alert and causes them to fight the unknown particles
- An inflamed, irritated leaky gut that cannot absorb vitamins, and minerals properly, thus taking us back to the top of this list

There is a dietary protocol called The Specific Carbohydrate

Diet that many people swear by. The diet consists of no grains and very specific sugars like honey and bananas that the intestines can rapidly assimilate. This diet has helped many people recover from Crohn's disease, Irritable Bowel Syndrome, and other intestinal disorders. The reason it works is because it removes all offending foods that either feed unwanted bacteria or require intensive amounts of enzymes to be digested until the gut can heal. The prognosis is usually to stay strictly on the diet for one year, at least, to see improvements.

Another diet that could potentially heal the gut is the Paleo Diet. The Paleo Diet consists of meats, vegetables, and fruits—no grains, processed sugar, or dairy—on the premise that this is what our ancestors ate for millions of years before grains were introduced. Interestingly, most scientists pinpoint the time grains entered our diets to be about 10,000 years ago. The university researcher who wrote the first book on eating "Paleo" is Dr. Loren Cordain, a Professor in the Department of Health and Exercise Science at Colorado State University in Fort Collins, Colorado. Dr. Cordain's studies on the diets of ancient hunter-gatherers show that they survived on mostly meats, berries, and plants. He believes that grains, dairy, and sugar cause a high-glycemic load on the body which leads to a host of other diseases such as diabetes, cancer, and intestinal disorders.

Dr. Cordain is absolutely right. The Standard American Diet (SAD) is full of processed sugars, dairy, and genetically modified grains that wreak havoc on the human body. However, I disagree with Dr. Cordain that we should avoid grains completely. Whole, organic, and genetically unchanged grains are good for the body and have many vital nutrients that are needed for human health. The problem lies in the fact that without proper soaking beforehand, these grains require a lot of enzymes to be digested. Unfortunately, our digestive enzymes are being used up at a rapid pace. Our bodies cannot keep up with demand. Allow me to illustrate the problem.

Currently in America it is common to eat toast or cereal with milk for breakfast, a sandwich with cheese for lunch, and pasta with cheese for dinner. Are you noticing a pattern? The common combination of milk and bread, bread and cheese is enjoyed all day long, day after day. Quesadillas, pizza, grilled cheese sandwiches, and cheesy garlic bread are all just variations on the same theme. We usually eat these things without any vegetables and call it a meal. Pizza tastes great and vegetables, well—don't. We already know the high gluten content in wheat grown in America is a known appetite inducer and is positively addictive. No broccoli stalk can compete. Put a bowl of vegetables next to a grilled cheese sandwich and just see which gets eaten first.

The Real Problem

The unfortunate truth is that it takes A LOT of enzymes to break down our hybridized high-gluten wheat flour—especially when paired with lactose-containing dairy products needing a host of lactase enzymes in their own right. The pancreas bears the brunt of this heavy job. It produces the enzymes protease (to digest proteins), amylase (to digest carbs), and lipase (to digest fats) and pumps them into the small intestine through the duodenum. The pancreas also produces the hormone insulin which specifically regulates blood sugar. In order to produce these enzymes the pancreas needs adequate amounts of vitamins and minerals that our current dietary choices no longer provide. We are not supporting our digestive system in its all-important job. Instead of placing deposits in our digestive bank account, we are constantly making withdrawals on our body's ability to produce enzymes. Day after day, we unknowingly pull from our body's nutrient reserves until one day there is nothing left. Our intestines can no longer digest foods and assimilate nutrients properly to send to the rest of the body, and a host of problems start to creep in like unwanted weeds in a garden.

Anciently, people ate more vegetables, good fats and whole, unadulterated grains out of necessity. They didn't have access to processed sugar, rancid fats, or adulterated milk. They didn't have to fight against the addiction of super-tasty processed foods because they didn't have access to them.

Currently we have easy access to all the sugar we can consume. And it's not just table sugar that we eat, but all the white flour and processed, stripped grains that turn immediately to sugar in our intestines. Sugar stresses the pancreas which has to produce more insulin every time your mouth sends a signal that something sweet (even if it isn't real sugar) is coming down the pike. With our diets becoming more and more processed food and sugar-based, you could think of your pancreas as being on constant high-alert or in "fire-drill" mode. Pancakes with syrup, a soda at lunch, a candy bar in the afternoon, ice cream after dinner day after day demands that your pancreas work harder and harder with fewer and fewer raw materials. Realize that the pancreas is fighting TWO fires: the first is the need for insulin to regulate blood sugar and the second is the need for vast amounts of digestive enzymes every time you eat poorly. If you are eating the Standard American Diet, I can assure you that your pancreas needs a break.

On the flip side, vegetables have natural enzymes that support and enhance the body's own digestive enzyme production. Vegetables also provide vital minerals and nutrients the body needs to produce its own enzymes. Eating fruits and veggies supports and lifts our own digestive powers to adequate production levels. Vegetables are preferable over fruits only because they are low in sugar. If you have a choice between the two, always choose more veggies than fruits. But if choosing between an apple or candy bar, obviously choose the apple.

Constantly eating hybridized wheat and homogenized, pasteurized dairy products depletes our enzyme-production system rapidly. I call this downward spiral The Double Whammy. "Double" because we hurt ourselves in two ways when we eat poorly: no supportive enzymes and nutrients from veggies plus the need for increased enzymes to digest our cheesy bread equals a double draw on the body's reserves. "Whammy" because this double dip on our reserves eventually whams our digestive system into sickness and disrepair.

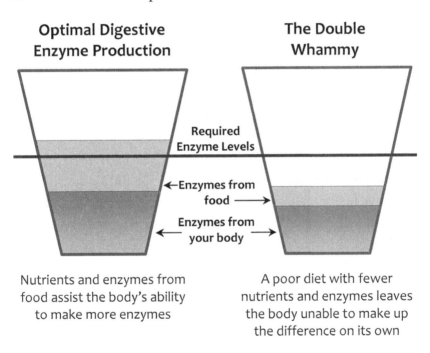

Optimal Digestive Enzyme Production

The Double Whammy

Required Enzyme Levels

←Enzymes from food →

←Enzymes from your body →

Nutrients and enzymes from food assist the body's ability to make more enzymes

A poor diet with fewer nutrients and enzymes leaves the body unable to make up the difference on its own

The simple solution to our current dietary mess is to vastly reduce the amount of processed foods, breads, sugars, and dairy and increase our consumption of healthy fats, vegetables, and easily digestible proteins. If your body isn't too far into disrepair you may be able to tolerate brown rice, quinoa, teff, and amaranth as well. If you struggle with multiple health issues, your intestines may need a break from all hard-to-digest foods such as grains and dairy. By giving the pancreas a much deserved break, we will improve our body's ability to make enzymes and keep the body in good repair.

The Body's Little Cleaners

Enzymes also have another function within the body: the metabolic enzymes are the late-night cleaning crew. After digestion is done for the day, metabolic enzymes go throughout the body and clean up messes and toxins. Enzymes break down these unwanted particles and escort them out of the body. These hardworking substances also fight inflammation of the joints and other body tissues.

Notice the phrase: "after digestion is done for the day," in the above paragraph. When is our digestion done for the day? Are we eating small meals with lots of vegetables and taking vitamins for trace mineral support to support our enzyme production? Or are we eating heavy meals with lots of enzyme-draining foods that our body will have to work on all night just to break down? This nightly cleaning can only occur if we have the raw materials and energy left to focus on cleaning.

As a mother, I know there have been many nights I chose to let the dinner dishes "wait until the morning" because I didn't have the energy to tackle them at night. I know your pancreas and other enzyme production systems probably feel the same way. Your personal energy levels mimic the energy levels of your internal digestive organs and digestive system. The two are inextricably intertwined. If you give your digestive system small meals with enzyme-supporting foods throughout the day, you will see your energy levels rise dramatically. This will occur because the system will have enough excess energy to "clean-house" and re-energize at night.

A researcher canvassed a group of women who were all doing a detox diet. The particular diet detox consisted of drinking vegetable juices and having a few small meals each day for 10 days. Participants reported increased energy across the board, and interestingly, many of the women reported an urge to do a very specific task. That task was consistent among the women and completely unknown to other participants. The unifying task: de-cluttering their homes. As their minds cleared and their energy increased, they felt a desire to get rid of things that were cluttering their lives. Could it be the outward manifestation of an inward cleansing?

I personally undertook a 21-day detox challenge to regain my health. I had been sick for so long I decided I had to do something drastic to turn the tide. The detox consisted of consuming a vegetable-based juice four times a day (every 2 hours) and one meal of cooked, non-starchy vegetables. I also had to take digestive enzymes with every juice or meal. Was it hard? YES. Was it worth it? Absolutely.

Before I started the detox I suffered from extreme brain fog. I had dealt with this problem for years and it was extremely debilitating. By 3 pm on the first day the brain fog was completely gone. GONE! My mind cleared and I could do everything I needed to do more efficiently. By the end of the first week, I could feel a connection with God again. By the end of the third week I felt better than I had ever felt in my entire life—even as a child. My mind and skin were clear, my belly was flat, and my energy was through the roof!

After the detox ended, I had no desire to go back to my old

eating habits. I drank vegetable juices often and had no desire for sugar or wheat. I trained for a half marathon and enjoyed balanced hormones and easy monthly cycles. I had great energy and could feel joy! I know it was the break from digestion, avoiding foods causing sensitivities, and taking additional enzymes that allowed me such a dramatic experience. It was then that I started to make the connection between enzymes and extreme health—as well as the gut and the brain.

But being human, my old eating habits eventually crept back about 6 months later and I started feeling "off" again. At that time, I didn't realize exactly what I needed to retain my health, as well as what I needed to avoid. In hindsight, one of the things I needed was to repopulate my intestines with good bacteria, known as probiotics, to strengthen and maintain the health gains I had earned.

Probiotics—the Defenders of Good Health

Probiotics are friendly bacteria found in our intestines. They give off waste that helps balance the intestinal flora and make the place hospitable to other friendly bacteria. We get our first exposure to these friendly bacteria right outside our mother's womb. As babies travel through the birth canal during delivery, they are exposed to these friendly bacteria and populate their own digestive systems. Breast milk then transfers more of these beneficial bacteria to our intestines where they grow and multiply to aid in our digestion and immune functions.

Recall the studies of Dr. Weston Price, who observed 14 extremely healthy groups of primitive humans around the world. One of the things each of these groups had in common was a natural source of probiotics in their diets from fermented foods. Each of these groups had healthy skin, teeth, hair, easy pregnancies and deliveries, and lived to old age without depression or dementia.

Researchers are now catching up with what Dr. Price already discovered: probiotics are ESSENTIAL to good health. They partner with enzymes and each other to break down food and make it easier to absorb nutrients. They are absolutely necessary for optimal functioning of the body and brain. They slow aging and protect the body against parasites, viruses, and toxins. And they are *crucial* to happiness, health, and vitality.

One of the greatest assaults on our probiotic population in our guts is the use of antibiotics—both by prescription and in the animal proteins we eat. Doctors have been prescribing antibiotics as a cure-all for many years. Unfortunately, when we take antibiotics, they kill the good bacteria in our intestines as well. In my early twenties, I was prescribed a low-grade antibiotic for many months to help battle acne. It was after being on these antibiotics long-term that most of my health issues began. I had never heard of probiotics and had no idea that I needed to assist and repopulate my intestines to maintain the good bacteria.

> Always make sure to eat properly fermented foods or take probiotics after a round of antibiotics—and do the same for your children. It is one of the smartest things you can do can do to ensure good health, both now and in the future.

Industrially raised animals are fed low-grade antibiotics to keep them protected from bacterial outbreaks. Unfortunately, these antibiotics are also found in the final product at your grocery store. This constant influx of antibiotics affects the probiotics in your intestines. Look for organic animal proteins or those raised without antibiotics for the sake of your intestinal health and balance.

Our other huge problem today is that the Standard American Diet (SAD) contains almost zero probiotic sources. We are currently getting no support from our diets unless we are going far out of our way to seek out probiotics on our own. Sources of natural probiotics from the healthy primitive groups were from lacto-fermented foods such as beet kvass, kimchi, sauerkraut, and properly-fermented yogurts. Lacto-fermentation allowed foods to ferment, or pickle, into a form that would allow long periods of preservation and thus, be available during scarcity. Lacto-fermentation does not strip foods of their nutrient content, but instead enhances the nutrient absorbability and provides the intestines with beneficial bacteria that produce lactic acid (which aids in digestion).

The closest thing our SAD has as a source of probiotics is yogurt. Unfortunately this yogurt is usually fermented from pasteurized, hormone and antibiotic-laden milk which is then complemented with an extra-heavy serving of sugar. Sugar feeds bad bacteria and fungi in our gut and throws our entire intestinal balance out of whack. Furthermore, because of the lack of enzymes in our milk sources due to pasteurization, digesting any milk product puts a heavy strain on our enzyme-producing organs. However, fermenting raw milk with a proper bacterial starter can produce a yogurt that is kinder to our digestive system. This kind of fermentation partially breaks down lactose and predigests casein—a protein found in milk that some find hard to digest. For more information on how to achieve proper lacto-fermentation, please see Sally Fallon's book *Nourishing Traditions*. It is filled with knowledge every person who feeds others should be privileged to have.

Probiotics are yet another example of the Double Whammy. We are not getting enough of them in our diets and yet are constantly exposed to sources of antibiotics. We eat foods that feed their enemies. Sugar, processed foods, and a lack of fiber put our intestines into a state of war that supports unwanted viruses, parasites, and fungi (especially candida). We are being very unfriendly to our poor, overworked internal probiotics. We need to cut out the bad stuff and include more supportive foods into our diets.

Probiotics are best gotten from perfectly fermented foods. However, realizing you are busy and may not have the time or interest to re-create the process of making perfectly fermented foods, I implore you to take a probiotic supplement *every single day*, without fail. Seek out a probiotic that has as many varied strains of bacterium as you can find in at least a 25 billion strain count. The reason you need this supplement every day is because the probiotic populations die out without constant assistance. This is mostly because it is hard to keep our probiotics happy without large amounts of good fiber in our diets. The SAD is notoriously low in good fiber. Sources of fiber that probiotics like are raw chicory root, Jerusalem artichokes, raw dandelion greens, raw garlic, and raw leeks and onions. I realize that few of the items listed are common in our diets and therein lies the problem. Change your diet to include as much plant fiber as you can and take your probiotics every day. Think of yourself as the general who is sending in back-up troops to the intestines. It is an act of love for your hard-working army. Do not leave them to defend you without assistance!

In summary, enzymes and probiotics are the keys to good health. They keep us young, make us look great, balance our hormones, enhance fertility, and keep our minds sharp. If you live in America, I can almost guarantee that your diet is not supporting healthy enzyme production or retaining the probiotics you currently have. By all means, change your diet to include more fruits, vegetables, and lacto-fermented foods. And as a backup plan, take a digestive enzyme supplement with meals and take probiotics every day. Your body will love you for it.

Chapter 9

THE TRUTH ABOUT FATS:

The Good, the Bad, and the Ugly

I grew up in Alabama near lots of family and lots of good food. When we would go to reunions in Tennessee everyone would bring a dish. We had fried okra, fried chicken, dressing (stuffing), ham, turkey, buttered rolls, casseroles galore, macaroni salads, giblet gravy, green beans with fatback, mashed potatoes with at least a cup of butter in them, deviled eggs, pecan pie, chess pie, chocolate pie, banana pudding, coconut pie, lemon cream pie, chocolate cakes, and other dessert delights. Our potlucks defined the term "comfort food."

My grandmother had a large garden to the side of her house. She would can okra, tomatoes, and other surplus vegetables every summer and share them with us. She and Papa also raised cows in their pasture across the road from their house. When my brother and sister and I would come up from "the city," we would help Papa feed his livestock. We would ride in the back of a truck full of alfalfa and push off sections for groups of hungry animals. My grandpa's cows were able to roam the land freely and eat grass and hay. My grandmother's freezer had fresh ground beef and steaks ready to be cooked at all times. I remember the beef from her house always tasted different than that from restaurants and the grocery store.

I realize now that my Papa's farm-raised beef tasted different because of what his cows ate, as compared to industrially raised cows that were fed corn. When cows eat corn it changes the fat ratios and content in their bodies. Looking back on my childhood, I realize now that I had access to both the best and worst fats available. The best were from the grass-fed cows and butter, while the worst fats came from trans-fat laden junk foods and snacks.

Realizing hindsight is 20/20, in this chapter you will learn what took me four decades to finally understand. You will learn why healthy fats are crucial to fertility, brain health, and vibrant cells. I will also reveal which fats are actually healthy and why there is so much confusion concerning this topic.

The Ugly

In the 1950's, a scientific study came out which pinpointed saturated fat and cholesterol as the causes of heart disease. Within a few years margarine became a staple in every American kitchen. It was touted as "better than butter" because it was cholesterol-free. Margarine made in these decades was made from vegetable oils turned into a trans-fat. Trans-fats are partially hydrogenated vegetable oils that become solid at room temperature. This occurs when an extra hydrogen molecule is chemically added to an existing fat compound in a lab or processing plant. Partially hydrogenated fats extend the shelf life of processed foods and made baked goods flakier. Foods fried in trans fats were crispier and lighter and seemed to taste better, too. Trans fats were used often back in those days. It wasn't until decades later that people started to understand the connection between trans fats and heart disease.

The ugly truth is that trans fatty acids increase your LDL cholesterol and decrease your helpful HDL cholesterol. They cause hardening of the arteries, heart disease[28], and increased obesity from inflammation[29]. They are also linked to an increase in type 2 diabetes[30]. In 2010, the state of New York approved an amendment forcing eateries and food carts to phase out trans fats to less than 0.5 grams per serving. California then outlawed use of any trans fats in the preparation of restaurant meals and baked goods.

Apparently, trans fats are enough of a health threat to require political intervention and most consumers have been adequately warned to avoid them. Unfortunately there is one caveat you need to know about. The FDA allows any food that has less than 0.5 grams of trans fats *per serving* to be labeled as having 0 trans fats. So if you eat 3 servings of a processed food that had 0.4 grams of trans fats per serving (while its label reads 0 grams trans fat), you would eat 1.2 grams of trans fats—without even knowing. The FDA agrees individuals should consume less than 1.0 grams of trans fats per day. Even that amount can lead to inflammation, weight gain, and heart disease. In this instance you must check food labels to know for sure.

As a voice of warning, any and all foods that have the words "partially-hydrogenated…" on their ingredients list should be avoided. This is the key phrase that indicates trans fats are lurking within their product.

The Bad

Many people have heard of trans fats and how they should be avoided, but most people don't realize that the amount of vegetable oils we eat on a daily basis is far more than is good for our bodies. If you eat at restaurants, buy snack foods at convenience stores, and consume packaged and bottled food, you are getting poor fats in large amounts. Even worse, the fats that are GOOD for our bodies have been labeled as ones to avoid. Let's dive deeper into why this is so.

First, a quick primer on types of fat:

- **Saturated fats** have all available carbon bonds occupied by a hydrogen atom. Because every carbon bond has a hydrogen atom on the end, these types of fats do not easily go rancid. They are very stable and are solid at room temperature. Examples of saturated fats are lard, butter, animal fats, and tropical oils. Your body can also make saturated fats from carbohydrates.

- **Monounsaturated fats** have two empty hydrogen atoms and are relatively stable. Our bodies make monounsaturated fats from saturated fats and use them for various purposes throughout the body. The oils from olives, almonds, pecans, cashews, peanuts, and avocados are examples of monounsaturated fats.

- **Polyunsaturated fats** lack four or more hydrogen atoms and contain omega-6 fatty acids (with two double bonds) and omega-3 fatty acids (with three double bonds). Our body cannot make these fatty acids and as such, they are labeled "essential". Polyunsaturated fats remain liquid, even when cold. The missing hydrogen atoms at the end of the double bonds make these oils highly reactive and they go rancid easily. These oils should never be heated or used for cooking. Soybean, corn, cottonseed, safflower, and sesame oils are examples of polyunsaturated fats.

Fats are also described by their length:

- **Short-chain fatty acids** have four to six carbon atoms and are always saturated. These types of fatty acids have anti-microbial properties and defend the body against bacteria, viruses, and yeast. These fats are less likely to cause weight gain than commercial vegetable oils because short-chain fatty acids are directly absorbable for quick energy. They are found in butterfat from cows and goats[31].
- **Medium-chain fatty acids** have eight to twelve carbon atoms and are found in tropical oils and butterfat. These fatty acids also have anti-microbial properties and can be utilized by the gut for quick energy like short-chain fatty acids. In addition, these fatty acids strengthen the immune system[32].
- **Long-chain fatty acids** have between 14 and 18 carbon atoms. Both omega-6 and omega-3s are long-chain fatty acids and have 18 carbon atoms each. Several other highly beneficial fats fall into the long-chain fatty acid category: stearic acid, oleic acid (the main component of olive oil), palmitoleic acid (strongly microbial and found almost exclusively in animal fats), and gamma-linoleic acid (GLA). GLA is found in evening primrose and borage oils and is often prescribed by naturopathic health practitioners to stabilize the monthly hormone cycles of women. Little wonder—GLA is used in the productions of prostaglandins which are hormone-like chemicals that are used within the cell for a myriad of processes. Scientists are currently researching and uncovering new functions of prostaglandins throughout the body.
- **Very long-chain fatty acids** have 20 to 24 carbon atom connections. Some of these particular fatty acids are

necessary for prostaglandin production, while others play vital roles in the function of the nervous system. **Interestingly, some people can manufacture these fatty acids from essential fatty acids, while others cannot. Those who struggle with this conversion usually had ancestors who ate a lot of fish and therefore lack an enzyme necessary to create these very long-chain fatty acids. The fish contained the fats in the required form so that the conversion wasn't necessary. These people *must* obtain these crucial fatty acids from egg yolks, butter, liver, and fish oils.**

Now that you understand the different types and lengths of fats, let's talk about the "scientific advances" of man on fat consumption in our diets.

As previously mentioned, starting in the 1950's, scientific research began to emerge that claimed saturated fats and cholesterol cause heart disease and should be minimized in the diet. Eventually eggs were labeled public enemy number one. Butter was then vilified for having both too much cholesterol and being full of saturated fats. Later, consumers were told that all fats were bad and Americans everywhere jumped on the low-fat diet bandwagon.

All this information from the powers that be has caused complete confusion among consumers everywhere. One day eggs are terrible for you and the next they protect against prostate cancer. Lard was used by every cook in America but once the fear of cholesterol emerged, processed lard (which was full of trans fatty acids) became the only fat cooks would use in their kitchens. We used to eat butter on a daily basis, and now dieticians tell us to use margarine spreads (no longer with trans fats, but softened polyunsaturated vegetable oils). Which fats are we supposed to eat? And even more importantly, who says we should eat them and why?

An eye-opening book by T. Colin Campbell titled *The China Study* explained more fully how nutritional research works within the realms of science, government, and industry. Dr. Campbell started his distinguished career in the 1970's and did research on mold toxins affecting children in the Philippines, bone density on women in China, a study on biomarkers for breast cancer, and went on to spend over 2 decades on a study of lifestyle and diet factors on disease mortality in China and Taiwan. Over the course of his career he was asked to join many boards and committees to assess the validity of nutritional claims for the good of the general population.

Towards the end of the 1970's, public interest and awareness of health studies and the claims of nutritional supplements and fad diets had increased. Dr. Campbell was invited to contribute to several groups comprised of scientists, researchers, and government experts to determine what guidelines should be disseminated to the public. He reports in his book that special interests were protected, truth and logic were ignored, and the power of influence was retained at all costs at the expense of the health of every consumer who believed these "expert" recommendations[33].

Dr. Campbell's research and experience led him to believe that a diet high in animal products led to cancer and obesity. However, others on one board he served with did not agree with him despite evidence supporting his claims. Those who disagreed with him also had consulting jobs and friends in the commercial egg and dairy industries. I was expecting Dr. Campbell to report obvious bribes and payouts to those in power by the aforementioned industries. What I learned was worse: your knowledge of what to eat and what not to eat was easily influenced by a single consulting contract here or an above-board first-class vacation perk there.

Additionally, what you have been taught about diet and fats for the past 40 years was also easily influenced by "the good-ol'-boy network" who simply watched each other's backs (and personal interests) to maintain positions of power through the creation of personal relationships. Scholars and scientists were influenced by the fear of losing their jobs or being discredited by fellow researchers and "experts" if they did not follow the status quo. Apparently, it was quite easy to defame one's research and findings by simply doing a smear campaign on their character or background. This led to a fall from popularity and eventual demotion or expulsion from the job or board. It reminded me of losing status in junior high or Hollywood—similar places where popularity is fickle and temporary.

We must also take into account the huge budgets certain industries have to promote their continued importance. For example, in 2003 Dairy Management Inc. had a budget of $165 million to "increase demand for U.S.-produced dairy products[34]." You can be sure that marketing has an effect on the perceptions of the public. If asked today if milk is good for you, most people will quickly respond, "Of course!" They will know nothing of the true effects of pasteurization, homogenization, or how a cow's diet affects milk quality. They will know little about how the cow was raised or treated. They will also be blissfully unaware of the history of milk consumption among different populations which might indicate one should avoid milk altogether. But does any of that matter when milk is accepted by the public as universally healthy?

The bottom line is this: the Adversary has been working on every man and woman to choose evil since the dawn of time. He uses fear to control and manipulate the masses. Fear of losing one's credibility, job, power, influence, and friends is a mighty productive tool against the dissemination of truth. If minions of the Adversary can get those in power to release dietary recommendations based on skewed data, it will only further the pain and suffering of many. I personally take any dietary recommendations released by scientists, "experts," or the government with a grain of salt. There are simply too many powers vying for influence.

So who can you trust? Yourself. Do your own research. Use logic, reason and sound judgment. Read research from alternate sources to counterbalance the voices of "experts". Assess how money or influence from large industries might be used to sway results. Humbly pray for discernment. Listen to your heart. With time, the answers will become clear.

Knowing how scientific nutritional research works in the United States can open up a whole new world of confusion for the health-conscious consumer. Many years ago my husband shared a principle with me called the "signal to noise ratio." This ratio describes the level of desired signal to unwanted background noise. Scientists use it to measure electrical signals and express the measurement in decibels. Informally, however, the term is used to describe the ratio of useful information to incorrect or irrelevant data. In today's world, we are inundated with noise: Facebook, Twitter, the news, commercials, infomercials, celebrity gossip, pop-up ads, and more. Trying to sift through this constant barrage of noise to find a morsel of truth can be exhausting.

The signal to noise ratio applies to spiritual truths as well. To hear the signal of the Spirit, you must sift through the noise from your own thoughts and the distractions of the Adversary. It can be difficult and seem overwhelming. To hear the Spirit, we must quiet our minds through meditation, pondering, and prayer.

John Pontius wrote the most beautifully simple description of how truth is given to man in his book, Following the Light of Christ into His Presence, pg. 40, when he writes "Good comes from God. Evil comes from the Adversary. Questions and analysis come from within." He was summarizing his explanation of the different mental messages, or noise, we have to sift through. He explained that messages from the Spirit are usually short impressions like: Fast today, Turn here, Bring that, Call her. Messages from the Adversary are usually a litany of reasons why you should or shouldn't do something—you deserve it, it's totally natural, everyone does it, the kids are too tired, no one will listen, you can do it tomorrow, it's late. He points out that Satan's helpers have trouble dishing out only one lie and that usually there is a litany of resistance to any good prompting. Then there are our own thoughts that are usually in the form of questions or analysis: "I wonder if I should do this today? What would happen if I left this for later? Did she really mean that?" and are usually in the first person. With this explanation, perhaps you can judge each thought and its source with a different lens of discernment.

When we apply the "signal to noise ratio" concept to the scientific advances of nutrition, there are large amounts of noise (scientific studies based on poor assumptions or having an ulterior motive as to what the final research results show) when one is searching for the signal (truth). And in no area has conflicting research caused more damage than in the world of fats.

The smear campaign on saturated fats began when a report was released by a researcher and scientist named Ancel Keys that blamed saturated fats for the rise in deaths from heart disease in the United States. This report was based on results from a study of six countries' fat intakes versus death from heart disease. He noted that Americans ate more saturated fats and had more heart disease when compared to the Japanese. However, Mr. Keys did not compare lifestyle factors like smoking, stress, sugar intake, or exercise levels among participants. Furthermore, when data from 14 additional countries was analyzed, the correlation between fat intake and heart disease deaths was completely disproven. Unfortunately the die had been cast, and the scientific community accepted the original report's findings. It became part of the status quo among researchers and nutritional experts to hold saturated fats in disdain and suggest a diet lower in saturated fats. As of 2014, this belief is still widely held among the scientific community, doctors, and nutritionists.

Unfortunately, after hearing that saturated fats were unhealthy, Americans then simply replaced natural saturated fats with trans fat laden margarine and vegetable shortening. As we now have perfect hindsight, this was not a positive collective move. Once trans fats were shown to be dangerous the population moved to polyunsaturated vegetable oils like soy, canola, cottonseed, corn, and safflower. The problem is, these oils go rancid rapidly when exposed to oxygen and when heated to high temperatures (such as during frying) and create free radicals when consumed[35].

Free radicals are created from oxidation of cells within the body. They are highly chemically reactive and can wreak havoc inside the body if not properly controlled. They attack cell membranes and red blood cells and have been shown to cause cancer, tissue damage, and skin problems. Newer research links free radical damage to premature aging, Parkinson's, Lou Gehrig's disease and Alzheimer's[36]. The body combats free radicals with antioxidants, which are mostly found in saturated fats, fruits and vegetables, and to a lesser extent in nuts, seeds, meat, shellfish, and eggs. As you might guess, the average American diet is already low in antioxidants even before the additional need for higher intake to combat free radicals from polyunsaturated fatty acids. Most of our diets are sorely deficient in many necessary nutrients with antioxidants being but one subset.

Another victim of the noise from scientific research is that of cholesterol. Cholesterol is produced by the liver and is also found in eggs, butter, cheeses, oysters, shrimp, and meats that we eat. Cholesterol is the "mother" of all hormones, which we will discuss in a later chapter. Cholesterol has inherent antioxidant fighting power and protects cells against free radical damage. However, scientists have found a link to high levels of cholesterol and blocked arteries leading to heart disease. Doctors prescribe statin drugs to control cholesterol levels within their patients. Unfortunately, they are conflicted as to what exactly causes high cholesterol. If you remove eggs, meat, and dairy from your diet, tests show that cholesterol levels do not necessarily decrease. However, if one removes sugar, white flour, white rice, and other refined carbohydrates along with rancid fats from the diet, cholesterol does decrease. Why would this be? **Because the liver produces excess cholesterol when we overeat sugar and simple carbohydrates. In other instances, cholesterol floods the bloodstream when we eat free-radical infused rancid fats in order to protect the cells and artery walls from inflammation**. In the latter case, cholesterol just happens to have been at the scene of the crime when all it was trying to do is protect your cells and arteries. Talk about getting a bad rap!

Some truths to combat the noise of the "experts":

- Saturated fats protect the liver from alcohol and other toxins like over-the-counter painkillers.
- Short and medium chain fatty acids in saturated fats have antimicrobial properties that protect the gastrointestinal tract from harmful microorganisms.

- A study of fat content in clogged arteries showed that only 26 percent was saturated (as from butter) while over 50 percent was polyunsaturated (as from soybean and canola oil)[37].
- Saturated fatty acids make up at least 50 percent of our cell membranes and are necessary for the cells to function properly. Cholesterol assists cell membranes to have necessary stiffness and stability, and along with saturated fats create and support cell integrity.
- Cholesterol is a precursor to estrogen, progesterone, and testosterone as well as corticosteroids which allow the body to deal with stress and protect cells and artery walls.
- Vitamin D production must be preceded by cholesterol. Vitamin D regulates hormones, reproduction, insulin, muscle tone, and growth.
- Bile salts which digest and assimilate dietary fats are made from cholesterol.
- Nursing mothers produce milk rich in cholesterol along with a special enzyme enabling babies to use it properly. Cholesterol is necessary for proper brain and nervous system development.
- Cholesterol supports proper function of serotonin receptors in the brain.

To discern more truth from all the noise, I began to analyze what happens in nature and how animals eat and live. There is no diabetes or cardiovascular disease in the animal kingdom unless they are nourished and overfed by humans. Animals seem to know intuitively what they should eat, when they should eat it, and when to stop eating. Animals give birth and propagate their species year after year, with zero assistance or "higher learning" required. I wondered what foods humans ate in the past that allowed us to stay strong, healthy, and vibrant and how humans knew they were good for consumption. Further research confirmed that humans have been eating wild and pastured animal products full of saturated fats for millennia without the problems found in modern-day hospitals[38].

I also began to look back into my own ancestry and how my parents, grand-parents, and great-grandparents ate and lived. All of my relatives ate lard, butter, eggs, and raw milk usually straight from their own pasture-raised farm animals. They ate vegetables straight from the garden and meat from the farm animals they raised. My father's grandmother lived into her late nineties. Her own mother was over 106 years old when she died. They lived in Tennessee and the Carolinas and we can trace our lineage back to Yorkshire, England, 1200 A.D. It is likely our ancestors there ate dairy (as the Neolithic British farmers were one of the first people to raise and cultivate cattle) as well as fish from the coast of Britain.

On my mother's side, my grandmother contracted Type 1 diabetes in her late teens. I witnessed her giving herself daily insulin shots for years. She lost all her teeth by her late sixties and eventually lost both her legs from the knees down. In spite of all this, she lived to be 77. She also ate lard and butter, vegetables straight from her garden, and meat from her farm animals. The one difference in her diet that I witnessed first-hand was a diet with large portions of white bread, biscuits, and sugary desserts. My mother's side of the family has a history of heart problems, diabetes, and skin cancer. They are also the family from which the amazing food arrived at our family reunions I mentioned at the beginning of this chapter. If you will notice in the list of foods, desserts played a large part in our celebrations, as well as fried foods, rolls, starchy vegetables, and side dishes. The food always tasted amazing, but I noticed we have what you might call a "portion problem" in our family.

My Papa taught me at an early age how to pack my plate full to bursting. Papa was a farmer and worked hard all day long. He could afford to eat larger servings (me as a young city kid, probably not so much). He instructed me to push helpings of mashed potatoes to the plate's edge so I could get more baked beans, casserole, ham, and rolls on the plate. Desserts required a whole plate by themselves. Both courses were washed down with full-sugar sodas. From reading studies and organizing my own observations, I realized it is highly probable that overeating sugar, white flour, and polyunsaturated oils are the cause of most of the diet issues in America today—not saturated fats.

The Good

From assessing the research of numerous sources on fats and human health, the signal became clearer and clearer while the noise began to fade away. **Your body knows what to do with saturated fats**. It has known how to handle these fats for millennia. The lives of your ancestors depended on them. Not only does the human body know what to do with saturated fats, it needs them desperately along with their high vitamin A and D content and microbial properties to protect and create hormones and other essential products within the body. What's relatively new to our diets are chemically processed vegetable oils, industrially raised livestock (raised indoors and fed genetically modified corn instead of grasses), excess sugar, stripped grains, and processed foods made shelf-stable with preservatives created in labs. These new introductions to our diets have replaced much needed nutrients with bad science and industry-led hype.

Another point to consider is that the human brain is 70% fat. The fats you eat determine the quality of the cells in your brain. Do you want to build your brain with rancid, chemically altered fats—or do you want to build your brain with the same substances that allowed the 14 primitive tribes Dr. Price discovered to live long lives and avoid depression and dementia?

If processed vegetable oils are not good for us, you may begin to wonder why they are found everywhere. They are used almost universally for frying, baking, and in salad dressings in homes and restaurants alike. The answer to this question is: money. Vegetable oils are cheap and easy to process. In addition, there are lobbyists who support the vast industry of edible oils in the United States. These industries have worked long and hard to gain market share and the public's trust while natural saturated fats and tropical oils have been vilified and shunned. No wonder so many of us are confused as to which fats to eat!

To reclaim your health and the health of your family you need to replace the new with the old. The best fats you can eat are those our ancestors ate: butter and lard from grass-fed, pastured livestock; eggs from free-roaming chickens who eat insects and seeds; extra virgin olive oil; coconut and palm oils; and fats from fish and fish livers.

If you get nothing else from reading this book, please remember this: *change the fats that you eat and you will change your life.*

Yes—butter from pastured, grass-fed cows is good for you! Way better than anything produced in a lab or factory. Lard from pigs allowed to roam in the sun has high levels of vitamin D and is a stable fat when cooked at high temperatures. Eggs from free-roaming chickens have higher levels of vital omega-3 fatty acids. Coconut oil has medium chain fatty acids that are proven to protect the body from microbes and bacteria (especially candida, or ist). Cod liver oil is an "old-wives tale" that proves to be true: it protects the body from free-radical damage and assists in brain and neurological development as well as hormone production.

Put butter on your vegetables. Pop your popcorn in coconut oil. Use real lard for pie crusts and occasional frying. Make your own salad dressings with extra virgin olive oil. Bake with coconut oil and butter. Take cod liver oil in a pill (it tastes gross, let's be honest). Consume eggs with the yolks which hold crucial nutrients not available in egg whites alone. Enjoy all these things in moderation and as long as you do not have a sensitivity or allergy to the food.

The brand of cod liver oil currently suggested by the Weston A. Price Foundation to have the most beneficial, unadulterated ratio of Vitamin A to Vitamin D is Green Pasture's Blue Ice High-Vitamin Fermented Cod Liver Oil which can be found online. My favorite, however, is the Fermented Cod Liver Oil plus High Vitamin Butter Oil in a capsule by the same company. Taking it caused my immune system to strengthen, my mind to clear, my body to handle stress better, and my food sensitivities to diminish. Check out www.westonaprice.org for more information on healthy fats.

Please note however, you do not need large amounts of these fats to satisfy your body's requirements. Fats are not meant to be the largest part of our diets. We need QUALITY, not sheer quantity. And let me be clear: a whole-food, plant based diet is the best kind you can adopt. But it is crucial to have some healthy fats along with those plants. And if and when you do eat meat, do it sparingly and make it count. Purchase only the highest quality available.

Also note that several researchers have found that once cancer overcomes a group of once-healthy cells, it feeds on fats (among other things)[39]. If you are diagnosed with any form of cancer it would be wise to cut out fats until the cancer is gone. See the endnote for the book titles and research of these men who were ahead of their time.

Some Guidance and Guidelines

Pay particular attention to the source of your fats. The reason red meat is tied to higher rates of heart disease is because of the corn that is fed to the cattle. Cows ate grasses for millennia before humans thought feeding them corn would help them get fatter, faster. Corn does make cattle grow fat, but not in a way that is positive for human consumption. Referring back to Dr. Campbell's *China Study* where he deduced that animal products were unhealthy for human consumption, I want to inquire as to the source of animal feed and living conditions of the animals his subjects consumed.

Cattle fed and finished on grasses has a wonderful balance of Omega 3 and Omega 6 fatty acids (Make sure the packaging says "Both grass fed and finished," otherwise they may feed very little grass to the cows and finish with corn). If cattle is fed corn, however, the Omega-6 content of their meat increases, and the Omega-3 content decreases, which has been shown to cause inflammation in humans upon consumption.

Liver meat and bone broths from grass-fed animals is full of crucial vitamins and minerals in an easily assimilated package. Also know that butter from cows feeding on rapidly growing spring grasses yields an exceptionally nutrient dense butter high in vitamins and minerals especially needed by pregnant and nursing women.

Egg-producing chickens need to have access to sunlight, bugs, and seeds to get proper nutrients and fat content into their eggs. The best eggs I've ever tasted are from chickens fed organic, gluten-free feed with access to the outdoors. Eat only wild-caught salmon that has fed on its natural diet. Its flesh will naturally be a deep pinkish-red and full of omega-3s and precious minerals. Be aware: manmade fisheries are now raising salmon fed corn and other ingredients that are not part of a salmon's historic diet. The flesh of these fish is a pale pink (some are even dyed darker pink and labeled accordingly) and the fat and nutrient content of the fish is sure to be different from its wild-caught cousins.

How animals are fed and treated determines the quality of the fat they provide. Humans have relied on these high-quality fat sources throughout history. We are not smarter as a species because we have "experts" telling us what we should eat. We are not better-fed because mankind has figured out how to raise animals faster on poor quality food. We are being manipulated by marketing and advertising campaigns and have to make a conscious effort to tune-out the constant noise all around us.

I have found the best sources for meats, eggs, and lard to be at my local farmers' market. I live in an area which is ahead of the game when it comes to naturally-sourced high-quality animal products. If you can, support your local farmers and get to know them and what they feed their animals. Your input matters. Consumer demand is impacting what products are being offered both at farmers' markets and in grocery stores. I have noticed many positive changes occurring that will impact lives for the good.

Perhaps most importantly, educate yourself and your daughters on the fact that these recommended fats are absolutely *essential* to healthy reproduction, pregnancy, and child development. Numerous studies have shown that saturated fats and cholesterol, along with the high levels of vitamin A and D they contain, prepare and sustain the body's need for high levels of hormones necessary for reproduction and breast-feeding. As mentioned previously, cholesterol is crucial for infant brain and neuron development, as well as cell formation and integrity.

Remember: Change the fats you eat and you can change your life and the lives of those you love!

Chapter 10
THE THREE NUTRIENTS ALL WOMEN DESPERATELY NEED

I could take you on a long, lengthy tease about what nutrients we desperately need with evasive and annoying marketing tactics. But because women needed this information yesterday, I'm going to get right to the point.

Nutrient Number 1

In today's world, you need Vitamin A like nobody's business. It is Nutrient Number 1 in importance and potential for deficiency. If you are sick, depressed, stressed, or infertile, I can almost guarantee you are deficient. I can almost hear you say: "What? I eat carrots, sweet potatoes, and some leafy greens. I take vitamins. I get plenty of Vitamin A!" Unfortunately you have been sold a lie. Beta-carotene is not the same thing as Vitamin A.

Beta-carotene is a *precursor* to Vitamin A. Your body has to convert beta-carotene to Vitamin A using fats, Vitamin E, thyroid hormone, and enzymes. So let's recap: What is the Standard American Diet deficient in? Good fats, enzymes, vitamins, and thyroid supporting minerals, that's what. Seeing as how many of us with poor health are low in these raw materials already, a Vitamin A deficiency can be the inevitable result. And that is even though, according to science, we're getting plenty of Vitamin A from carrots and other vegetables. Excessive Vitamin A deficiency can create blindness, night blindness, conjunctivitis, dry hair, ridges on fingernails, reproductive issues, and weaken the immune system. But what if you merely hover between having low Vitamin A and having an extreme deficiency? You get depression, infertility, weight gain, toxicity, and a lack of ability to deal with stress without the other markers of Vitamin A deficiency. You get overwhelmed easily, pull away from social interactions, and constantly second-guess yourself.

What Vitamin A Does

- Vitamin A is necessary for digestion of proteins. The quickest way to deplete yourself of Vitamin A is to eat a high-protein, low-fat diet.
- Vitamin A is needed to assimilate calcium. Vitamin A is found in the fats in milk (according to the Dairy Council, www.milk.co.uk, a one cup serving of whole milk contains about 9% of an adult's recommended daily allowance), but little to no Vitamin A is found in low fat and nonfat milk. Drinking skim milk depletes our Vitamin A stores in the liver. Atherosclerosis is caused from calcium deposits in the arteries. Joint issues are caused by poorly directed calcium deposits. Without good fats and Vitamin A to instruct our bodies how to use calcium, it ends up in the wrong place.
- Vitamin A gives stem cells direction on what kind of cell to become in developing fetuses. Heart tissue, liver tissue, and intestinal tissue all get their instructions from Vitamin A.

A lack of Vitamin A can cause organs to be malformed and can be the cause of miscarriages.

- Vitamin A is necessary for proper skin, eye, and bone formation.
- Vitamin A is required to make T-cells in the immune system.
- Vitamin A is required for EVERY hormone created in our bodies including: cortisol, DHEA, estradiol, and testosterone. These hormones are all converted from cholesterol using Vitamin A and other enzymes. Insufficient Vitamin A means impaired hormone production.

What Depletes Our Vitamin A Stores:

- Vitamin A stores are rapidly depleted from STRESS. Do you have any stress in your life? Since Vitamin A is required to create cortisol, "the stress hormone," there is little wonder that women in today's world are rapidly depleting their liver stores of Vitamin A and are highly likely to be deficient.
- Fever and illness deplete Vitamin A. Make sure to give children cod liver oil, liver meat, or liver pate when recovering from illness, or blindness can result.
- Pharmaceuticals like acetaminophen and a host of prescriptions must be metabolized in the liver using Vitamin A.
- Pesticides require Vitamin A to be broken down and removed from the body.
- Physical exertion depletes Vitamin A as extra minerals are used to repair cell turnover.
- Dioxins in smoke and pesticides exhaust Vitamin A.

Do you see the pattern? **Vitamin A combats stress and toxicity!** Without enough of it, you will be chronically stressed, toxic, and run-down. Since today's world is full of toxins and stress, we desperately need to be aware of our Vitamin A intake and replenish our stores after stressful situations. With a good store of readily available Vitamin A you need not worry about the overwhelming abundance of toxins around us or stressful situations taking you out of the game of life.

Why Are We Deficient?

Just a generation ago, mothers served beef or chicken livers on a regular basis. Children consumed milk and butter from pastured, grass-fed cows. Chickens were allowed to roam in the sun and eat bugs and seeds along with their chicken feed. Mothers through the ages have fed their children cod liver oil—much to the disdain of the children's taste buds, I am sure. All of these factors led to diets full of easily assimilated Vitamin A. Nowadays, people don't consume liver because we have been told it is toxic. We disdain butter because it has lots of cholesterol and is "fattening." Eggs come in and out of dietary popularity and most people have been taught to drink low fat or nonfat milk. I don't know anyone who feeds their children any source of cod liver oil.

I have a hunch that many of us cannot process Vitamin A from beta-carotene, even if we ate a perfectly healthy diet (which we don't). Note that those with diabetes, poor thyroid function or a poorly functioning liver cannot assimilate beta-carotene well, if at all. There are certain populations that cannot process lactose in milk because it wasn't a part of their diets historically. It takes hundreds if not thousands of years for the human body to express a genetic tendency that is carried through to every generation from natural selection deaths. Because we have modern medicine, it is highly unlikely people with an "undesirable" gene will die before having children of their own. Therefore, it seems likely that if your ancestors had a history of easily accessible Vitamin A through fish and fish livers if they lived by the sea, or animal liver if they lived inland, that these ancestors may not be able to convert Vitamin A from carotenes easily if at all. And this inability will be passed from generation to generation.

So what do we do? We will do ourselves a huge favor by eating foods that contain fat-soluble Vitamin A in a ready-to-use form. Vitamin A in this form is found in whole-fat dairy, organ meats (liver, giblets) and fish livers—especially cod liver oil. I was not exposed to eating organ meats very often growing up but know that my parents and grandparents were. My grandparents lived to their seventies and eighties. One grandparent is still alive at 87 and has a great memory. I fear that our society's drift from eating organ meats and taking cod liver oil is affecting the health and fertility of generations to come.

If nourished properly, children develop strong organs that set the foundation for a healthy life. One study done in Norway showed that cod liver oil fed to babies in their first year of life had a direct effect on lowered diabetes levels throughout their lives when compared to the normal population[40]. It is highly probable that the powerful fat-based nutrients in cod liver oil allow a strong foundation as the pancreas is growing and forming that prevents diabetes later in life.

Also note that babies and children CANNOT assimilate Vitamin A from beta-carotene, nor are they capable of storing Vitamin A effectively. They simply do not have the capability yet. Feed your little ones butter, cod liver oil and small amounts of organ meats regularly. They will thank you for the rest of their lives.

The amounts of easily assimilated Vitamin A found in chicken and beef liver are astounding. Do not believe the myth that liver is toxic and should be avoided. Eaten in moderation, and with a sufficient amount of vitamin D in your body, the body assimilates the nutrients found in organ meats beautifully. I suggest buying liver from trusted sources at your local farmers' market. Knowing the people who raise the animals you eat gives you the opportunity to ask what the animals were fed and how they were raised. Shortening the distance between farmer or rancher and your table can make a huge difference in the quality of food you eat.

DO KNOW THIS: Vitamin A and Vitamin D work harmoniously with each other and protect one from too much of the other. If you have sufficient amounts of Vitamin D in the body (approximately 1000 IU per day), you will not be in danger of Vitamin A toxicity and vice versa. The proper ratio according to The Weston A. Price Foundation is 10 parts Vitamin A to 1 part Vitamin D for optimum absorbability. That translates to 10,000 IU of Vitamin A and 1000 IU of Vitamin D per day for adults and half those amounts for babies and children. This fact leads us to our next sorely needed Vitamin: Vitamin D.

Nutrient Number 2

Lately, the nationwide Vitamin D deficiency issue has gotten big press. But do people really understand the issue? There are a number of confusing points on the subject of Vitamin D that need to be addressed. I hope that after you understand them, you will make sure you are getting the proper amounts in your diet and especially in the diets of your children.

What Vitamin D Does

- Vitamin D allows calcium to be absorbed from food and supplements. For years, women were told to take extra calcium to prevent osteoporosis, but the bigger problem was actually Vitamin D deficiency. Just like Vitamin A, D is required to tell calcium where to go. Without both of these components, calcium can end up in the wrong places.
- Vitamin D is necessary for nerves to communicate properly with each other.
- Vitamin D is required for good muscle tone and healthy skin along with proper growth and bone density.
- The immune system requires Vitamin D in order to fight against bacteria and viruses.
- Vitamin D is a crucial component of a healthy reproductive system and is especially important during pregnancy and lactation.
- Vitamin D is necessary for the production of chemicals in the brain that create stable moods and give one a sense of well-being as well as protect us against depression.

Where is Vitamin D Found?

While researching sources of Vitamin D, I found a government website that claims "very few foods naturally have vitamin D." Then the website continued to list a few paltry items like fatty fish, beef liver, and mushrooms that have small amounts found within them. Wild caught salmon and mackerel have decent amounts of Vitamin D (500 IUs and 230 IUs per 100 gms respectively). The website did not mention that shrimp is high in Vitamin D, nor did it mention lard from pigs with access to the sun (Yes, you once again have the green light to use lard).

We've been taught that Vitamin D can be produced within the human body if we get enough exposure to the sun, and this is true. However, the sun must provide UVB rays with sufficient intensity to provide the building blocks for Vitamin D. One problem we have is that in the mid-latitude of the United States, the sun is only intense enough to provide these building blocks between 10 am and 2 pm during the summer months. As women, we also have a tendency to slather on sunscreen every time we walk outdoors for fear of aging prematurely. Succinctly put: We are not getting enough Vitamin D from the sun through our haze of sunscreen and sun avoidance during the "most damaging times of the day," nor are we eating fatty fish in sufficient quantities. We are likely getting most of our Vitamin D through fortified milk (if you can tolerate it) and other fortified foods. We are most likely deficient in this critical vitamin.

So how did people get Vitamin D in decades past? People worked outside and never used sunscreen. They ate more fish and fish liver oil. They fried things in lard and used lard in recipes. Pigs store Vitamin D in their fat cells just like humans. Of course, pigs must have access to the sun in order to do this. If you find a good source for lard, make sure it is from pigs that are not raised indoors.

It is interesting to note that our ancestors did not all perish from skin cancer even though they never used sunscreen. Here's the truth: your body can protect itself from the sun with enough antioxidants and good fats—we just aren't eating properly. Omit rancid fats, white flour and sugar. Eat more fruits and vegetables straight from the tree or garden. Get more good fats, more A, D, K, and other essential nutrients in your diet and DITCH THE SUNSCREEN. Sunscreen has tons of chemicals that your body has to break down through the liver (thus, draining your Vitamin A stores). Unless you seek out the world's cleanest and chemical-free sunscreen brands (which are just now starting to appear in custom boutiques, but not big box stores or drugstores yet), you are denying yourself of Vitamin D and putting a huge toxic load on your liver. Many of the chemicals in sunscreen are known hormone disruptors like phthalates and lauryl sufates. Don't think that things you put on your skin do not have to be broken down. They all end up inside the body and have to be eliminated.

Certainly if you're going to be out in the sun all day, protect yourself in the shade, don rashguards, wear hats, or use a minimal amount of sunscreen. But please reconsider slathering it on your kids' entire bodies before they step outside. Remember, all things in moderation. Feed them better food with more nutrients to combat the negative effects of the sun, and let them enjoy the sunshine and benefits of Vitamin D.

Your least time-consuming source of Vitamin D is D3, cholecalciferol, in a supplemental liquid form. Each drop of Vitamin D oil usually contains about 1000 IUs. The recommended daily allowance is 1000 IUs, but if you are deficient and depressed, between 5000 and 10,000 IUs is usually prescribed. Make sure you have sufficient Vitamin A in your diet to aid absorption and assimilation of large doses of Vitamin D. Over 10,000 IUs of Vitamin D taken orally on a daily basis can cause toxicity. Sunlight never causes Vitamin D toxicity because your body will simply stop converting the raw materials when it has stored its limit.

For the record, the kidneys have to process Vitamin D to its active form. If your kidneys are sluggish or clogged, you will have problems manufacturing and maintaining proper Vitamin D levels. To keep your kidneys in top form, avoid sodas, coffee, taking calcium without fats, and make sure to get enough B6 in your diet. Another crucial mineral for kidney function is our Nutrient Number 3.

Nutrient Number 3

Our average American diet is pathetically low in many nutrients, but one of the most vital gets very little airplay. We hear a lot about calcium, but very rarely do we hear about calcium's counterpart, magnesium. Magnesium is the fourth most prevalent mineral in the body and is usually stored in the bones and tissue. Getting a decent read on your body's stores is rather difficult for this reason.

What Magnesium Does

- Where calcium strengthens and tightens, magnesium loosens. Magnesium is the magic mineral that relaxes muscles and tension.
- Magnesium is required for over 300 enzymatic processes as a cofactor.
- Magnesium is required to regulate nerve and muscle function.
- Blood pressure and the rhythm of the heart rely on magnesium to stay in healthy ranges.
- Magnesium is instrumental in regulating blood sugar.
- Proper immune function requires magnesium in readily available amounts.
- Magnesium is essential for proper hormone functionality during menses and pregnancy.

Where Do We Get It?

Magnesium is found in halibut, spinach, black beans, almonds, peanuts, and lots of other vegetables, beans, whole grains, meats and milk. Unfortunately it is only found in small amounts in each one of these items. That means that to get the magnesium you need, you must eat a diet rich in whole foods—*all the time.* Forget the white flour, white rice, sugar, sodas, and processed foods. If you eat any of the just-listed pseudo-foods you are missing the opportunity to feed your body magnesium containing foods. And since processed foods are designed to thrill the taste buds, while whole foods simply nourish the body, sometimes making the right choices and getting enough magnesium just doesn't happen.

Over the years, it is likely that the body will pull magnesium from the bones to make up the difference. Our bones are rich sources of mineral stores but they are not meant to be consistently depleted from a diet poor in essential minerals. They are meant to support the structure of the body and stand as a mineral back-up plan in desperate times. When you eat mineral deficient foods, you are signaling to your body that you are in desperate times. It is likely that a deficiency accumulates over the years and begins to cause problems with digestion, monthly cycles, fertility, moods, memory, blood sugar, and the immune system.

Humans need about 350 mg of magnesium each day. One of the easiest ways to "catch up" if you're feeling tense and deficient in this powerhouse mineral, is to take a bath with Epsom salts. Epsom salts are magnesium sulfate crystals and were named after Epsom, England, where they were first dissolved in water and used as a health aid. Use 2 cups of Epsom salts dissolved in hot bath water and soak for 20 minutes. You will feel relaxed and calm afterwards as the magnesium is absorbed through the skin.

I also suggest you take a magnesium supplement at night to make up for all the poor dietary choices that may have happened throughout the day. Magnesium helps you fall asleep soundly. For maximum absorbability internally, make sure to buy magnesium citrate, glycinate, or aspartate as magnesium oxide and sulfate were found to be less absorbable by the body[41].

What About Other Nutrients?

Replacing the top three missing nutrients cannot help you heal and recover without the availability of every other necessary nutrient in the body. No vitamin, fat, or mineral works alone. I sometimes think of humans as individual cells in a larger body created perfectly by God. Some of us are gifted at creating or entertaining, others are amazing at organization and cleaning, while others are great at leading and inspiring. But no one works alone—no one. Everything we do is with, through, and for others. From doing copious amounts of nutritional research I've realized that nutrients are the same way—they all interact and depend on the presence of other nutrients.

For example, Dr. Weston Price discovered that no matter how abundant minerals are in our diets, without Vitamin A and other fat-soluble vitamins, these minerals cannot be absorbed and utilized properly. The fat-soluble vitamins found in butter, raw-milk, eggs, and fish are keys that open the locks to our cells and instruct them how to use minerals properly. We need these vital keys to have healthy brains, neurons, temperaments, and normal sexual development[42]. Healthy fats are the mortar to the bricks of vitamins and minerals. One without the other does not build a strong house. In fact, you could imagine that every time you eat poor fats you are building part of your brain and other tissues with weak mortar.

Is it any wonder that occurrences of Alzheimer's disease are rising at an alarming pace? These people are the first generation to reach a substantial age after eating poor fats and being exposed to ever-increasing toxins for much of their lives. The lack of healthy fats to make up the brain tissues and protect them against toxicity is taking its toll. The mortar in the cells of their brains is crumbling and their minds are being lost in the process. The loss of these incredible minds and memories is devastating not only those that love them, but to the world.

I cannot stress this enough: Make sure you change the fats in your diet to those eaten historically by humans and explained in the chapter on Fats. You will see improvements in memory, mood, fertility and overall health in both you and your children.

For vitamins and minerals, the best multivitamin I have ever found is USANA's Essentials pack. For the record, I do not sell USANA vitamins nor do I receive any endorsements from them. I recommend them only because they have made me feel significantly better. I started taking USANA vitamins in my early twenties after my best friend convinced me of their quality and effectiveness. Several years later I quit taking them out of laziness. My health deteriorated after I stopped taking them but I never connected the cyclical depression and problems handling stress with vitamin consumption.

Years later I stumbled upon an independent publication that ranked dozens of supplements for bioavailability (how easily assimilated they are in the body). USANA got a score of 98% out of 100. They blew away the competition. They also seem to be ahead of the game in adding helpful trace nutrients like Co-Q10 and n-acetyl l-cysteine that aid in brain function and capacity. Realizing this, I began taking the Essentials again in 2011.

In 2012, I was lucky enough to meet with one of their top chemists/biologists and got to interview him on many topics. I was very impressed with his concern for others and the depth of his knowledge of nutrient requirements for women (and more specifically, woman trying to become pregnant). For me, knowing who is in charge of developing and maintaining products I use gives me a much greater degree of confidence in using them. I wholeheartedly recommend taking the mega-antioxidants and chelated minerals found in the Essentials set. I take mine twice a day with meals to increase absorption. Usana is a multi-level marketing company but you do not have to become a distributor to purchase items. You can buy the products directly from their website at www.usana.com.

Something else to note about multivitamins is that they never contain enough calcium or magnesium. I have checked numerous brands, both for adults and children's dosages, and they are often in the 2-15% RDA range. Do not think that because you are taking a "multi"-vitamin you are getting enough of all the nutrients. You must get calcium and magnesium in addition to your multivitamin.

Another nutrient you must supplement separately is iron. If you suffer from fatigue, get your iron levels checked. Women often suffer from anemia unknowingly. Anemia occurs when the body has low red blood cell levels often from a lack of iron in the blood. It can exhibit itself as fatigue, malaise, and difficulty concentrating. Iron also affects your body's ability to utilize thyroid hormones. From personal experience, getting your iron levels corrected can result in a dramatic increase in energy and your overall sense of well-being.

Many of you may need additional support and information

found in the next chapters. Increased knowledge and understanding is crucial to combat the onslaught of our next topics: thyroid problems and toxicity.

Chapter 11
THYROID ABUSE:
How to Stop the Cycle of Neglect

Sitting like a delicate butterfly wrapped around your esophagus lies one of the most underestimated organs in your body. A powerhouse of productivity, it ranks among the most important when it comes to maintaining your vitality and happiness. Conversely, its performance failure can perpetuate misery and sap strength. This vital organ is the thyroid.

Like most of the important organs within the body, we remain blissfully unaware of our thyroid until something goes wrong. Unfortunately, symptoms of thyroid malfunction are often vague, imprecise, and leave the affected party at a loss as to the source of their problems. Depression, weight gain, fatigue, brain fog, and hair loss are just some of the random symptoms of an imbalanced thyroid. Sadly, symptoms like these are on the rise—especially among women.

In this chapter you will learn what the thyroid does, what it needs to function properly, and the real reasons why it begins to break down. You will also learn why the medical system misdiagnoses thyroid problems and what you can do to protect and heal yourself and those you love.

Thyroid 101

Your thyroid produces two substances called T3 and T4 which signal to other cells to produce proteins or increase oxygen usage. Translated, T3 and T4 regulate your metabolism and energy levels. Your pituitary gland produces a substance called thyroid stimulating hormone, or TSH, which stimulates the thyroid to increase or decrease T3 and T4 production based on blood level readings. Adjacent to the thyroid gland are the parathyroid glands which independently regulate calcium levels in the blood. The thyroid, pituitary, and parathyroid are all crucial to achieving balanced levels of energy and oxygen usage within your body.

Most problems with the thyroid can be traced to either too much or too little thyroid hormone. If your body isn't making enough, the situation is called hypothyroidism. Hashimoto's thyroiditis, an autoimmune disorder where the body begins to attack its own thyroid tissue, is an example of one cause of hypothyroidism. Symptoms can include:

- Depression
- Dry skin
- Cold hands and feet
- Fatigue
- Easy weight gain
- Difficulty losing weight
- Hair loss (especially the outer third of the eyebrows)
- Slow pulse
- Brain fog
- Constipation

If your body makes too much thyroid hormone, such as with Grave's disease, the situation is labeled hyperthyroidism. Symptoms can include:

- Rapid pulse
- Pounding heart
- Anxiety and jitteriness
- Unexplained weight loss
- Diarrhea
- Trouble sleeping
- Rapid-fire thinking, or a speeding up of brain processes

The thyroid is part of the essential triangle of hormone production performed by the endocrine system. The thyroid, ovaries, and adrenal glands create hormones that are essential to human survival and reproduction. If one point of this triangle is weakened or fails, the other two try to pick up the slack. Unfortunately in today's world the thyroid is usually the first to falter for several reasons. Lack of nutrients from poor nutrition or reduced soil quality is the first offender. The second are the toxins we must break down and eliminate every day.

Your thyroid needs iodine in order to function properly. The terms T3 and T4 actually refer to how many iodine atoms are attached to the final chemical structure of the thyroid hormone. Without enough iodine the body struggles to make these essential substances. Iodine is found in saltwater fish, seaweed, cow's milk, milk products, and iodized salt. The recommended daily intake of iodine is 150 mcg for anyone over four years of age. Make sure you are getting at least a minimum of 150 mcg of iodine daily for optimal thyroid functionality.

Selenium and zinc are two vital minerals that affect the uptake and usage of thyroid hormone. Without supplementation, zinc intake is noticeably low in the standard American diet. Zinc deficiency affects enzyme function and the uptake of thyroid hormone while a selenium deficiency affects the production of thyroid hormone itself. Selenium is supposedly more readily obtained but if farm soil is not replenished with minerals between plantings you may be getting less than you think. The RDA for zinc is 8-11 mg per day for adults and the RDA for selenium is 55 mcg per day.

Iron is also necessary for proper assimilation of thyroid hormone. Iron is required for oxygen transport between cells. If iron levels are low, the cells cannot properly respond to the orders given by thyroid hormone. Requirements for adult women are 18 mg per day while men only require 8 mg per day.

With all these nutrient requirements just to make thyroid hormones, you may have realized that an unintended deficit could have disastrous results. Small deficiencies can add up to big problems over time. Your safest plan of action is prevention. Food is always the best source of nutrients for the human body. If you have access to perfectly clean and nutritious food sources take advantage of them. If you're not sure about your food sources, make sure to take supplements.

As for the second offender, toxin removal, we will discuss toxicity in detail in the next chapter. For now, know that selenium is a key ingredient for toxin removal and the more toxins your body has to eliminate, the less selenium is available for your thyroid. Robbing Peter to pay Paul in this case may very well be the reason that so many people suffer from thyroid problems.

A Cautionary Tale

In 2004 I took a leap of faith and went to a hormone clinic to try and figure out what was causing my health problems. Back then, these clinics were rare and unproven. Today, they exist in every major city. Women are more open to trying alternative therapies as a way to find their path back to health. Luckily for me, I landed in a quality establishment with great doctors. And while I was there I learned, for the first time, about the thyroid gland.

As the doctor went through my blood test results, he pointed out one thing in particular. It turns out that I was making antibodies to my own thyroid tissue, also known as Hashimoto's thyroiditis. He then pointed out that even though I had this disorder, my T3, T4, and TSH were all "within healthy range markers." I had been told this before. In fact, my blood tests always returned showing all markers being in an acceptable range. Regardless of the fact that I felt like death warmed over, nothing was showing up on standard blood tests as an indicator of ill health.

But this time the doctor did something different—he read my list of symptoms. He checked my pupils (they dilated very slowly). He looked at the dark circles under my eyes. He checked my cold hands and feet—and he *listened*. He listened to the litany of problems I was experiencing and then he did something even more amazing. He prescribed me thyroid medication in spite of the fact that I was "in the healthy range."

He explained that symptoms speak louder than any blood test. He also clarified that just because your thyroid levels are in an acceptable range according to science, you may still be out of an optimal range for your own body. If you could have taken a snapshot of your thyroid numbers when you felt your absolute best in life, you would have a great baseline for comparison when determining your current thyroid health. Unfortunately, most of us don't have that. So doctors rely on a scientifically determined "acceptable range" to tell them whether a person needs assistance or not.

Having suffered greatly from hypothyroid symptoms while never showing any thyroid hormone levels being "out of range," my heart goes out to all of you who actually fall outside the acceptable thyroid hormone level parameters. Thyroid imbalances can make your life absolutely miserable, and I send you compassion and empathy. But please know that a little thyroid medication and nutrient supplementation can do wonders in this area. You may just need to find the right doctor—and the right thyroid medicine.

There are two kinds of commonly prescribed thyroid meds. Armour thyroid is desiccated pig thyroid with naturally occurring T3 and T4 (along with slight levels of T1 and T2 but the function of these two substances is currently unknown). Synthroid or Levothyroxine (a synthetic, patented thyroid replacement pharmaceutical) is all T4 which the body then, theoretically, converts to T3.

Most people are prescribed the synthetic T4 version for thyroid assistance. But for some, it just doesn't seem to do the job. Others swear by Armour thyroid and insist that it is the only substance that works for them. I believe that having both options available to those in need is crucial. Armour thyroid is most likely the best default option because it contains both T3 and T4 and is the closest substance to human thyroid hormone. However, if you have Hashimoto's thyroiditis where you fight against your own thyroid tissue and hormones, Armour thyroid is too close to the human version and synthetic T4 is a better bet. If you struggle while taking only T4, you may need some supplemental T3 as well. Some available T3 sources are Liothyronine, Triiodothyronine, and Cytomel.

Flash forward four years to 2008. A new doctor found that I had a lump in my thyroid that needed to be checked. At the age of 35, my doctor said she had a 95% chance of getting to tell me that all was well. Unfortunately I fell into the unlucky 5 percent—the biopsy came back testing positive for cancer. I went into shock. Despite all my health problems I never thought I would be diagnosed with cancer. Especially not with two small children at home who depended on me.

You go through a lot of emotions when you contemplate the end of your life. To be honest, I wasn't thrilled at the thought of living a long life after struggling through my first 35 years. I knew my husband would be alright, but children need a mother. And the thought of leaving my own daughters motherless was heartbreaking.

So I fought back. And luckily, I won.

After extensive lab analysis on my full thyroidectomy showed the cancer was not an aggressive form and that all cancerous cells were contained within the removed organ, I breathed a sigh of relief. And six years later all is still well.

However, from this experience I learned something interesting from my thyroid surgeon. Dr. Reid Anders Rosendahl came highly recommended and had done hundreds of specialized thyroid surgeries in one of the largest cities in the country. He had seen thousands of patients and studied the thyroid in depth. He shared his hypothesis that the control group used to determine healthy thyroid levels must have included people who were unknowingly hypothyroid which increased the healthy average ranges of TSH as a result. TSH is the chemical that tells your body to produce more thyroid hormone. When it is high, you are not making enough. Currently healthy TSH levels are listed as 0.5 to 4.5. After all the patients he had seen and analyzed symptoms from, this surgeon felt that a more likely healthy range would be 0.5 to 3.0. He found that most of his patients felt significantly better with lower TSH levels than those at the top of the currently accepted range.

If his hypothesis is true and the healthy range levels were actually adjusted, millions of Americans could fall into this new unhealthy span of the scale. It is amazing to think how one re-adjusted scientific chart could suddenly justify the suffering of many and give them a true diagnosis.

The final thing I learned is this: the protein portion of gluten closely mimics thyroid tissue. If you have a leaky gut and become malnourished to the point your body begins to exhibit autoimmune disorders, and you contract Hashimoto's thyroiditis, wheat is no longer your friend. Through a leaky gut, gluten enters the bloodstream and triggers a resolute immune response. Antibodies then mistake thyroid tissue for gluten protein and the attack begins. People with Hashimoto's thyroiditis comprise 30-40% of all papillary thyroid carcinomas (a common type of thyroid cancer).

After my diagnosis of Hashimoto's I didn't know about the gluten connection. If I had eliminated wheat from my diet in 2004 I might have avoided cancer and possible death in 2008. I would have definitely sidestepped years of depression and anxiety regardless of the cancer. Please learn from my mistake and consider eliminating gluten from your diet if you have thyroid issues. Your body might then be able to heal itself and save you years of misery in the process.

Next we will discuss toxicity, the body's defenses against it and what your can do to protect yourself.

Chapter 12
TOXICITY AND YOUR GENETIC MAKEUP

It is no secret that the world we live in today is different than it was a few hundred years ago. We have car exhaust, factory run-off, cell towers, artificial flavorings and preservatives, fake sugars, off gassing, pesticides, weed killer, and chemicals galore. Never before have our bodies had to work so hard to remove all the unwanted substances we encounter.

Some of us were fortunate enough to have been born with top-notch toxin removal skills. But others got the short end of the stick on these removal capabilities. I lost the genetic lottery for toxin removal. It took me 38 years of depression, difficult pregnancies, hormone issues, insomnia, cancer, brain fog, and a host of other symptoms before I figured this out. If you struggle with depression and other health issues, this may be a factor for you as well. Make no mistake, how your body "takes out the trash" has a huge deal to do with your overall health and how you feel every day.

Genetics

Newer genetic research is uncovering the ways different genes predict how we process chemicals, break down hormones, and fight inflammation. Over the past ten years, scientists have made progress by leaps and bounds in this area. I had no idea these genes could be revealed and explained until a wonderful doctor decided we should run my genetic panel to try and decipher what was going wrong.

A simple blood draw and $425 later yielded some fascinating results. I share the following results with you for discussion points with your doctor. You can get this test run on your own, but you will likely need someone well versed in the medical field to explain them to you fully. This test and many other helpful analyses are found at Genovations website, www.gdx.net. These results opened a whole new world of understanding of why depression and illness are more likely in some of us than others.

Within the body are Phase I detoxification enzymes which start the toxin breakdown process. They are then followed by Phase II detoxifiers to finish the job. The Phase I processors are labeled the CYP-genes indicating the cytochrome P-450 system. Polymorphisms (or less than optimal genetic construction) in any of these genes indicates a potential decrease in your enzymatic abilities—meaning, your enzymes do not efficiently break down toxins into substances that can then be converted in Phase II detoxification and removed from the body.

I have two polymorphisms in this area. One is in an enzyme that breaks down estrogens and one is in CYP3A4 gene which detoxifies over 50% of all prescription medications and most steroid hormones. From past experience, I had learned my body does not deal well with certain anesthesias and prescription painkillers. Recovering from surgery took me weeks just to get out of bed, where others were up and going the next day. Morphine and Demerol did not lessen pain but instead, made me feel worse. Having the understanding of why your body should avoid certain pharmaceuticals could allow you to avoid painful situations and long recoveries.

Phase II detoxification takes the substances altered in the Phase I process and prepares them for final elimination. There are several categories in Phase II such as: Methylation, Acetylation, Glutathione Conjugation, and Oxidative Protection. If you have problems with methylation, your body has a compromised ability to break down neurotransmitters like dopamine, epinephrine, and norepinephrine. Acetylation processes detoxify environmental toxins like tobacco smoke and car exhaust fumes. Glutathione detoxifies solvents, herbicides, fungicides, and heavy metals. Finally, oxidative protection occurs through SOD (superoxide dismutase) genes which give the body enzymatic defense against oxidative stress like that from free-radicals.

Dr. Mark Hyman, the author of *The Ultramind Solution* and several other best-selling health books, has found that through years of helping patients regain their health that nearly all of his very ill patients have compromised glutathione activity. He calls glutathione the "Mother of All Antioxidants" and notes there are over 76,000 medical research articles on the subject of its importance in the human body. Glutathione is produced in the body and is exceptional at getting rid of free radicals and toxins. It is usually recycled in the body using Vitamins C, E, and selenium (which your thyroid also needs and competes for) and is used over and over again before being retired. That is, unless we become overloaded with toxins, or depleted of nutrients and the cycle breaks down. **He suggests that almost half of the population has a compromised GSTM1 or GSTP1 gene which indicates weakened glutathione function—and along with that, a propensity for illness and disease.**

Dr. Hyman has this genetic abnormality, as do I. If you suffer from illness, toxicity, and depression—you may have this genetic variation as well.

There are things you can do to help your body detoxify itself.

You are not foreordained to a life of illness and misery. You just need to know what those steps are. By taking action, you have a much greater chance to feel good and operate optimally. Following is a list of ways to boost glutathione function.

- Eat cruciferous vegetables like kale, broccoli, cauliflower, collard greens, and cabbage.
- Ensure adequate intake levels of Vitamin C, Vitamin E, selenium, zinc, and magnesium.
- Take L-glutamine as a supplement.
- Consume milk thistle (silymarin).
- Most importantly, you must have adequate levels of B1, B2, B6, B12, and folate in order to increase glutathione efficiency.

Note that you need Vitamins C, E, selenium, zinc, magnesium, B1, B2, B6, B12, and folate to improve glutathione production. What are we not getting enough of in the standard American diet (SAD)? All of the above nutrients. In order to re-start our detoxification channels, we are each going to have to replace the junk food and empty calories with whole foods. You cannot get enough magnesium and B vitamins unless you eat a super healthy and clean diet and, most likely, take supplements.

Considering commercial produce farmers may or may not rotate crops and add compost to the soil (both expensive and time consuming but necessary to replenish minerals to the land), we may be consuming less than optimal nutrition without even knowing it. On the other hand, vitamins and supplements are not the answer to a diet full of junk and bad fats. All the vitamins in the world will not help you fight off a constant lack of fiber and healthy fats found in the SAD. Remember: fiber, good fats, vitamins, and minerals all work together with the good bacteria in the gut to be assimilated into the body. It is an orchestra of functions that need all the players to create beautiful music. Do your best to supply the best raw materials to your body every day.

Some people today have started taking prescribed high-dose Vitamin B shots. The shots actually include several B vitamins and other nutrients to help absorption in the body. For those with depression, unrelenting pain, or consistent illness, you may need a boost to get your glutathione production back on track. One of my doctors experienced fatigue and pain so severe she could not work for years. After taking B shots for a year she began to recover and now runs a thriving practice. It is her personal belief that providing the body with much-needed B vitamins begins the healing process at the cellular level. These B shots are something you may want to discuss with your doctor.

There are several other areas of detoxification pathways besides glutathione. However, research seems to indicate that under-performing glutathione is the most widespread detoxification problem we have today. By increasing your glutathione function and efficiency you may be able to turn around your health problems with little further effort.

Toxin Avoidance and Removal

Possibly like many of you, I often feel like the canary in the coal mine. For those of you too young to know the origin of the phrase, here's the story. In previous times coal mines did not have ventilation shafts to draw out methane and carbon monoxide when hitting a new coal seam. Coal miners would take a caged canary into the mines with them to detect poisonous gases. If the bird stopped singing and died, the miners evacuated as fast as possible to avoid the same fate. The canary is the warning signal to others—the first indicator of imminent danger.

Because my body is extremely sensitive to toxins, I often feel like the warning voice to my family and friends. A warning can be a good thing. However, the best scenario is for you to have an optimized detoxification system so you don't have to worry about daily toxin exposure. But until you have perfectly rebuilt nutrient stores and detoxification pathways, I want to give you some helpful tips on things to clean up and avoid, some of which you may never have considered.

Heavy Metals

Metals like mercury, lead, cadmium, arsenic, and aluminum exist in the earth and in many of the useful things we use every day. The problem occurs when these metals somehow get into our bodies. Mercury exists in fillings in your mouth and in large fish, as well as fertilizers on our crops. Aluminum is found in our deodorant, pots and pans, and in foil around our food. Other metals show up in our water sources. These all end up in our bodies which are not designed to handle heavy metals. You need optimally functioning glutathione pathways to trap and remove these metals. Without them, these substances accumulate and wreak havoc on your gut, joints, and brain.

Some suggestions:

- Get a simple water filter for your tap water. Britta brand water filter pitchers work great and are economical.
- Know that traces of mercury have been found in high-fructose corn syrup—remnants of the manufacturing process. High-fructose corn syrup is cheap, plentiful, and commonly used by food manufacturers to sweeten many food items. It is found in sodas, ketchup, baked goods, powdered and bottled sauces, and other pre-sweetened

packaged foods. Check food labels carefully. Avoid it if possible and do NOT feed it to your kids. (Their developing brains are very delicate and susceptible to toxins.)

- Find a biological dentist and get your mercury amalgams (fillings) removed. Biological dentists should be trained in how to remove these fillings while protecting you from contamination in the process (visit www. iaomt.org to find a biological dentist in your area). This can be a dangerous process so make sure you are not ill, pregnant, or nursing and have found a dentist with excellent training and reputation. Studies have shown that chewing releases mercury vapors into your mouth which then travel to your gut and brain. This constant contamination could be causing a host of problems throughout your body. Mercury depletes glutathione and Vitamin C and inhibits B1 and B6 absorption. A lack of B vitamins is a known cause of depression. Mercury toxicity causes neurological disorders, speech problems, and has been connected to Alzheimer's, autism, and a host of other illnesses.

- If you suspect heavy metal exposure and toxicity, find a doctor who is well-versed in heavy metal detoxification. There are provocation tests that can show you exactly which metals are being held in your body. (I found I had serious levels of mercury and lead—which was not good news.) There are several ways to chelate heavy metals and remove them from the body but this should be done under a doctor's care. Releasing heavy metals into your bloodstream without raising the capacity for removal can be very dangerous. The research I did scared me away from taking action on my heavy metals toxicity for years. I wanted to find a natural, slow way to remove the offending metals, and I didn't have a doctor to help me in the process. With the above warnings being stated, one natural product I researched extensively and tried myself with good results was zeolite with humic acid marketed as Zeolite-AV. Research it and decide for yourself. And if you choose to take it, make sure your bowels empty twice a day and drink lots of water. You can find it online at www.zeolite.com.

- Get rid of aluminum pots and pans and do not use pans with non-stick coatings. Aluminum foil should not touch your food. Ceramic coated cookware is fine.
- Eat only organic produce whenever possible. Toxic heavy-metal laden refuse is turned into "fertilizer" and resold to conventional farmers who may or may not know its origins.

Mold

Mold in your home or workplace can sap you of vitality and health. Molds give off poisonous mycotoxins that overwhelm the immune system. They are often found in damp, moist areas that are hidden in our homes or offices. If you have unexplained fatigue, pain, and depression get a mold test done on your environment. You can find them at hardware stores. They are easy to culture from the air in your desired location, and then mail them in to be tested.

If your find you have been exposed to toxic molds, increase all the necessary nutrients mentioned earlier to empower your glutathione production. You will need extra amounts of these nutrients (especially zinc, selenium, Vitamin C, and B vitamins) to expel the mycotoxins from your body and recover your former health.

Candida

Candida is a commonly used name for yeast fungi found in the human gut. It is optimally found in perfect balance in the intestines. Unfortunately today we do not live in optimal conditions. Both mercury and mold mycotoxins along with antibiotics and a diet high in sugar and carbs encourage the overgrowth of candida albicans in the gut. The results are disastrous—especially in the female body due to hormone disruption. This problem is usually misdiagnosed by doctors and yields random and seemingly unrelated symptoms. This topic is so important that it will be discussed at length in its own chapter.

Parasites

I know, gross! Just the thought of nasty, life-sucking organisms living in your body can turn your stomach. Unfortunately the way we currently eat creates a perfect environment for these unwanted creatures to survive and thrive. They give off nasty toxins, rob you of vital minerals, and mess up your gut's ability to absorb nutrients. They can land in the intestines, liver, pancreas, and even your brain if left unchecked. And the vast majority of the time you don't even know they are there.

A diet high in sugar and low in good fats creates an environment in your organs that is very welcoming to parasitic invasion. Sugar feeds candida which can cause leakages in the gut lining (as do gluten, antibiotics, and other toxins) and a confused immune system. Poor fats provide the body with mediocre cell construction materials. This can then lead to trapped toxins within our cells that are welcoming to invaders. Say you unknowingly ingest a parasite egg from tainted produce which would normally be dissolved in the stomach or gut. Unfortunately, if you have a compromised intestine, the egg can find its way through to a weakened, toxic, overworked liver or other organ to "set up shop." With these first lines of defense crippled, invaders of many kinds have access to normally off-limit areas.

Dr. Hulda Clark, now deceased, wrote several books about disease and immunity. Her claims were based on the belief that ALL disease is caused by either parasites or pollutants in the body. She discovered that all living creatures have a frequency that can be determined with a frequency generator. She then went on to find that molds, viruses, bacteria, and parasites give off frequencies between 0 Hertz and 1000 Hertz. Humans resonate above this 1000 Hertz range. She created what she calls a "zapper" that sent out an electrical pulse through the body that stunned and killed anything in the less than 1000 Hz range. Many people swear by her zapper technology. Others claim it is a hoax of epic proportion. I've read her books and seen some of the testimonials of the zapper and my opinion is, don't be too quick to write her off. Read about it and decide for yourself. Her books can be found online. Additionally, her son created an online business offering clean herbal supplements and toxin free household items. His website is located at www.drclarkstore.com.

Dr. Clark also created a parasite cleanse protocol using natural herbs such as wormwood, green walnut hull, and cloves that are known to eradicate parasites. The protocol is available online for free, and the herbs can be found easily online or at local health stores.

Parasites can cause inflammation within the body which can keep you from losing weight or lowering your cortisol levels. If you suffer from un-diagnosed fatigue and depression, parasites could be the cause. In my opinion, it is worth an annual herbal tune-up to have peace of mind that there are no unwanted invaders in your body.

Pesticides

To get rid of unwanted pests on our food and in our homes, we often turn to chemical pesticides found on store shelves. We don't know how they were created or what they contain but we spray them around our homes and put them on our grass and shrubs and then in our gardens. For someone with optimal glutathione function, these chemicals may be easily removed. For the other half of us, you are adding a drop to the bucket labeled "internal toxic overload." It may not bother you while you are young, or even in your twenties or thirties, but eventually you start to feel rundown and don't know why. All pesticides add to your cumulative load. Some add cupfuls of distress and others just teaspoons—but they all add to the problematic bucket. Pesticides, unless they are made from organic matter that is not toxic to humans, are not good for our bodies, our food, or our environments. There are many natural ways to get rid of pests in the garden and in our homes. Check out www.naturalsolutionsbook.com for ideas on how to keep pests at bay without chemicals.

Household Chemicals

Like pesticides, household chemicals and cleaners add more stress to our detoxification centers. There are many items that fall into this category: paint thinner, lead-based paints (now illegal), new carpet off-gassing, foam mattresses and pillows, gasoline, gas stoves, dish soap, dishwasher detergent, clothes detergent, sink cleaner, counter cleaners, floor cleaners, oven cleaners, tub and shower cleaners, stainless steel cleaners, granite cleaners, and carpet cleaners. The toxic soup we allow in our homes is wearying to our bodies.

Some suggestions:

- Air out your house several times a week. Open the windows for 15 minutes, no matter what the weather. Some homes are built so air-tight that to save on heating and cooling bills, we are surrounded by stale and toxic air. Houseplants are also helpful in removing toxins from the air—get one medium sized plant for each big room and a small one for each bedroom.
- When cooking with a gas stove, always use the fan over your cooktop.
- If your home has an attached garage, park cars outside or crack the garage door to allow ventilation.
- Never store gasoline, lawnmowers, weed-trimmers, and the like in spaces that are attached to your home. Get an outdoor shed or use a detached garage. Same thing for paint thinners and other noxious household chemicals. (Or better yet, get rid of them!)
- Some old dryers have belts that have asbestos in them. Use your ventilation fan in your laundry room (I always wondered why it was there, too) as your dryer runs.

Most household cleaners are formulated by chemical companies that want to impress their shareholders with greater market share and big quarterly revenues. To do this, they spend lots of money on marketing ads and commercials so you think they are offering a great product. They test their products individually to ensure they are not dangerous to humans. However, when you add one cleaner for your toilets, another for your sinks, another for your floors, another for your tubs and showers, and another to dust, you may hit your personal toxic overload before your realize it. Like pesticides, these household cleaners each add their share to your toxicity overload bucket. You want to avoid these additional stressors at all costs. If you are already ill or depressed, get these chemicals out of your house!

I have searched high and low for good quality, safe cleaning products. Here are some of the brands I have found that do not irritate me or my family. This includes freedom from itching, coughing, and other skin, sinus and lung irritations. I do not receive any endorsement fees from any of these products. I just honestly love them.

- Norwex cleaning products—mops and specialized cleaning cloths that trap germs and viruses; also offer gentle,safe cleansers including laundry detergent, dishwashing detergent, and dishwashing liquid (www.norwex.com)
- Advantage 20X Multi-purpose Cleaner—all-purpose cleaner for floors, walls, countertops, and surfaces. Removes mold, mildew, grease, and grime. Comes concentrated so you can add water to make it the strength you need. (www.amazon.com)
- Silver Shield Sanitizer spray—all natural formula with colloidal silver to kill germs and protect the spread of colds and viruses. For use on doorknobs, toilets, keyboards, remotes, telephones, etc. (www.silver-botanicals.com)
- South Austin People Soap (So.A.P.)—bar soaps, liquid hand soaps, shaving bars, dog shampoo, and laundry detergent. I love this whole line. The laundry soap comes in unscented, tea tree, and eucalyptus, has no unwanted chemical residue (divine!) and is formulated for high efficiency washers. The jasmine-scented bar soap is fabulous, and the cherry almond liquid soap smells like heaven. I ditched my old shaving cream and use the Kaolin shaving bar instead with great results. The dog shampoo is a little

heavy on the patchouli for my taste but is great for our dog's fur and avoiding dog and human skin problems (our old dog shampoo had wheat gluten in it—which caused issues for me every time I put my face near our dog's fur). Prices are reasonable and I love the chemical-free results. (www.southaustinpeople.com)

Personal Products

As women, we use dozens of products on our skin every day. We usually don't even give them a second thought. Unfortunately, many of these products use preservatives and other ingredients that take their toll on our toxin removal system and our hormones. In small doses they may not pose a large threat, but to a compromised body or as a combined load, the effects can be disastrous. You must understand that every product you put on your skin must be broken down and removed through the body's interior trash removal system. Every single one.

Some specific product ingredients you need to avoid are: phthalates, lauryl sulfates, and parabens. These ingredients are linked to several types of cancer, hormone disruption, dermatitis, eczema, lower sperm count, liver damage, kidney damage, and eye damage—and they are found in the vast majority of the products we buy in our local stores. Skin products, hair products, and makeup have little to no governmental regulation over what chemicals they can use and then sell to the consumer. Now that I know more about these particular chemicals, I shudder when I think of our children using these products and the likely connection to rising infertility, depression, and cancer rates.

Unfortunately, you currently have to protect yourself through your own efforts. While other countries have laws against the use of certain chemicals in personal products, the population of the

United States is woefully unprotected. Fortunately there is an increasing amount of demand for clean personal products, and with a little research, you can find a plethora of great items.

Some products I use and have had great results with:

- Jose Maran Argan Face Moisturizer and 100% organic argan oil—I use the oil on my face and body as moisturizer (www.sephora.com)
- Tarte Amazonian clay 12-hour foundation and lights, camera, lashes! Mascara—the entire Tarte line is great (www.sephora.com)
- Silver Shield Deodorant, Silver Tongue Oral Disinfectant, and Botanical-C serum (www.silver-botanicals.com)
- Davines haircare products (www.amazon.com)

Another point to consider is personal hygiene products. If you use tampons, you are putting an absorbent material inside your body. Did you ever consider what was on that absorbent material? Cotton is sprayed with pesticides and other chemicals to keep bugs from eating the boll. Growing up in Alabama I saw crop-dusters flying frequently over cotton fields, spraying the land. I didn't think much of it back then, but now realize this sprayed cotton is what our clothes, sheets, and tampons are made of. The uterus is a terrible place to have toxins reside. Consider switching to organic tampons and give your body a break.

If you want to take things to a super level of "clean" here are some other things you may want to think about:

- Organic cotton sheets and clothing
- Organic mattresses and bedding (you spend a LOT of time in bed, 1/3 of your day!)
- Use only low or no VOC (volatile organic compounds) paint in your home

- "Green" carpeting and flooring
- Get a filter for your showerhead as well as your drinking water. Chlorine in our tap water is released as steam during hot showers. It is then absorbed through our lungs causing a host of problems. Drinking chlorinated water kills off good bacteria in the intestines.

Final Suggestions

In closing, I realize this information can be daunting to someone who is dealing with health issues. I suggest focusing first on supporting your body's detoxification pathways with good food, supplementation, and filtered water. Then focus on what products are in your home that you can change out quickly and inexpensively. Next focus on what you put on your skin. Finally, consider a long-range plan for the larger and more expensive items like bedding and mattresses.

By small and simple things, great things are brought to pass!

Chapter 13
HOW TO DEFEAT CANDIDA
Plus Bonus Detoxification Strategies

No conversation about toxicity would be complete without a discussion on candida. Millions of people suffer from the random symptoms that occur once this underhanded organism enters the scene. Doctors don't seem to recognize its indicators; and if they do diagnose candida properly, an uphill battle remains to eradicate it completely. The entire Western culture plays up to candida's strengths and leaves human bodies weakened and vulnerable to a hostile takeover as a result. If you do find yourself among the inflicted, candida is a fierce opponent and one on which you must educate yourself if you hope to evade its grasp.

Candida is a fungus which blooms when naturally occurring intestinal yeast are not kept in check because of an imbalance in the intestines. Good bacteria in the gut normally keep yeast from overproduction, but once these probiotic reserves are weakened the yeast can start to morph into a candida form. After a round of antibiotics, use of birth control pills, or use of cortisone or other drugs, what was once a harmless single celled yeast organism can morph into a multicellular rapidly reproducing invader known as candida.

Classic symptoms of yeast overgrowth are thrush, skin rashes, and vaginitis. However, you can have problems with candida within your intestines without any of these outward symptoms.

There are more than 150 species of candida yeasts, but only ten of these cause trouble for humans. The most common troublemaker in the human body is candida albicans. This type of candida sends out rigid roots called hyphae that can pierce intestinal walls and organs causing leaky gut syndrome and other serious issues. This invader feeds on simple carbohydrates such as sugar, white flour, fructose, honey, syrup, milk sugars, and other sweeteners as well as processed grains. Under perfect conditions, candida can double its population in *one* hour. As candida multiplies inside your intestines, it builds a protective biofilm that keeps your intestinal immune army at bay—all within 24 hours. If the biofilm is breached, candida has been known to alter its structural chromosomal arrangements to literally shape-shift into a more protected state. This fungi has been shown to produce seven different kinds of colonies to maintain genetic diversity and adaptability. This stuff wants to survive—and it wants you as its host.

Once candida has set up camp, it can multiply and travel to other parts of the body. In extreme cases, unchecked candida can cause death. For most of us, however, it simply causes misery, illness, and a chronically overworked immune system.

From all the research I have done, candida is a very likely source of much of the suffering women experience today.

Symptoms of candida include:

- Depression
- Migraines

- Food intolerances
- Fatigue
- Brain fog
- Anxiety
- Low sex drive or an extremely high sex drive
- Vaginitis
- Acne
- Eczema
- Cravings for sweets
- Fatigue
- Brain fog
- Mood swings
- Dizziness
- Poor memory
- Irritability
- Learning disorders
- Gas and bloating
- Sensitivity to chemicals and perfumes
- Thrush
- Acid reflux
- Chronic pain

The Standard American Diet which is high in sugar and processed foods and low in nutrients, good fats, and fiber, is the perfect diet to encourage candida. Candida converts sugars and processed grains into carbon dioxide and ethanol. Ethanol causes brain fog and must be broken down by the liver. The toxic by-products of candida begin to stress an already overworked organ and more toxicity builds up in the body as a result.

If you are one of the genetically challenged and are a poor producer of glutathione (as explained in the previous chapter), mercury build-up within the body can cause yet another problem.

Yeast can hold double their weight in mercury. As a strategic immune response, the intestines will allow yeast to grow in order to absorb mercury to keep it from reaching other parts of the body. In *The Yeast Syndrome* by Dr. J. Trowbridge, doctors specializing in candida treatment reported to Dr. Trowbrigde that 98% of their patients with chronic candida also had mercury toxicity. If you are sick and depressed, a very likely cause may be that you are full of toxins due to the inability to remove heavy metals and the inevitable candida overgrowth that results. Mercury must be removed from your system before candida can be ultimately conquered (see the previous chapter for tips on how to eradicate heavy metals).

Chronic stress also increases the chance of candida overgrowth. Stress causes sugar to be released into the bloodstream so the body can take flight quickly. The pancreas releases insulin simultaneously so the sugar can enter our cells and be used for fuel. This release of sugar into the bloodstream feeds candida and allows rapid regrowth. If under chronic stress, the pancreas becomes overworked and the adrenals have to attempt to restore balance. When the adrenals become overloaded, the immune system and our ability to combat candida are both compromised. Rapid overpopulation then leads to more toxicity and stress within the body.

Some researchers insist that candida is also the cause of hormonal imbalances. Toxins, excess sugars and mineral-poor diets change the pH balance in our intestines to become unfavorable to good bacteria and highly favorable to candida. Researchers say that candida can bind to hormone receptor sites, and is a known endocrine disruptor. From personal experience, I would have to agree with these findings. Clearing out candida was the best thing I ever did for my own hormonal balance—without exception.

Do I Have It?

There are several methods of determining if you have candida overload. The easiest method is to do a spit test and take a questionnaire. The candida spit test is done by placing a glass of water by your bed at night and upon waking, spitting into the glass. Allow 15 minutes to pass and then check the glass. If you have long, spindly webs trailing from the top of the water you have a positive indicator for candida. Dan at www.yeastinfectionadvisor. com has posted a questionnaire on his site that you can access to determine if your health issues may be caused by candida. Visit www.yeastinfectionadvisor.com/yeastinfectionquestionnaire. html to see if your score is above 200. He has found that a positive saliva test paired with a questionnaire score over 200 has a high rate of accurately detecting candida. He has worked with many candida sufferers over the years and can also guide you through the healing process. His assistance and advice is free. From my personal studies of many sources, his website pulls together an in-depth collection of solid research on the hows and whys of candida and can help you get started quickly. His free newsletters are also fantastic. Dan makes a living from selling supplements to combat candida through his site. But he sells only the best on the market, eliminating confusion and frustration for many.

Another testing source is the Comprehensive Digestive Stool Analysis from Genova Diagnostics. This test shows both desirable and undesirable bacteria in the intestines along with the amount (or lack thereof) found. If fungal numbers are high, a Susceptibility Profile shows which pharmaceuticals and which natural anti-fungals will kill the yeast in question. Make sure to request a Susceptibility Profile if you have this test run. This can be a life-changing piece of information, as not all invaders respond to every form of treatment. I highly recommend this test and profile because it will show you exactly what you can use to eradicate unwanted fungi specific to *your* body.

My doctor suggested this test for me and was surprised at the results. She stated she had never seen such high levels of candida—it was a clear cut case for candida overgrowth. However, my good bacteria levels were also quite high. I had been taking probiotics for years but apparently without the anti-candida diet and biofilm elimination, probiotics alone will not eliminate candida. The interesting thing was that in spite of high numbers indicating candida, I had no other classic indicators. I did not suffer from thrush, skin problems or any other outward manifestation. But inside, a battle was raging and my health was declining as the fight wore on. Please learn from my mistakes and consider candida as the source of your depression, hormone problems, and illness—even without any classic outward symptoms.

What Can Be Done?

The good news is that this invader can be evicted from your system. The bad news is that it is going to take some work. Of all the health solutions available to mankind, the removal of candida is one of the hardest to execute. It will require strict adherence to dietary changes, and one slipup could set you back quickly. However, thousands of people swear by its positive life-changing effects. They say it is worth every effort to be able to be free of depression, think clearly, have energy, and feel joy.

To remove candida from your system you must:

1. Follow a strict diet that will starve the fungi and prevent reinfection
2. Remove any biofilm in your intestines
3. Take anti-fungals

4. Heal the gut
5. Have an efficiently moving colon

First Step: The Diet

The anti-candida diet (ACD) is designed to starve the candida while feeding the human body. It is interesting to note that it is very similar to a Paleo Diet which promotes no grains, dairy or sugar. In addition to these restrictions, however, the ACD disallows yeast, vinegars, mushrooms, and fruits for a time. The initial phase of the diet lasts from 2 to 8 weeks and depends on how much candida exists in the body. The diet consists of non-starchy vegetables, clean meats, good fats, and some nuts and seeds. Potatoes are not allowed, and beets and carrots should be minimized because of their high-sugar content. After a 2 to 8 week period of strict dieting, you may start to introduce fruits and legumes slowly and watch for adverse effects. If all is well, you can continue with the new food additions. If not, you need to revert to the strict diet until symptoms subside and re-introduce new foods at a later date.

Things you can eat are: eggs, steamed veggies, guacamole, salsa (without vinegar), lemons, limes, parsnips, squashes, cold-water fish, olive oil, coconut oil, flaxseeds, arrowroot powder, grass-fed beef, chicken, and turkey. I'm not going to sugar-coat it for you; this diet can be very difficult. Many things must be made from scratch as nearly all condiments and dressings have vinegar in them. To succeed, you need to plan and shop ahead of time and always have something pre-made on hand.

You must avoid all kinds of sugars and sweeteners (except for Stevia and xylitol) as they feed yeast. It is crucial to success. It is also the hardest thing to give up. Sugar has been shown to be more addictive to the human brain than heroin. And sugars are found everywhere, including in good-for-you fruits. Plan for a period of discomfort as sugar withdrawals kick in. They will inevitably be followed by candida die-off symptoms called Herxheimer's which are similar to the flu: aches, chills, feeling down and depressed. The good news is all of this will be short-lived, followed by great improvements in mental clarity, energy levels, and sense of well-being. It will be hard, but it will be worth it.

Second Step: Biofilm Removal

One of the trickiest parts of candida removal is dissolving the protective biofilm these organisms create within the intestines. The biofilm itself is a polysaccharide matrix that acts as a protective shield against the intestine's immunity army. If the biofilm is not removed, anti-fungals will not be able to do their job.

The following substances have been shown to remove biofilm: monolaurin (from coconut oil), serrapeptase, N-acetylcysteine, selenium and lactoferrin. Dr. Junger, author of *Clean Gut* recommends 600 mg of monolaurin twice daily. His extensive experience with intestinal healing makes me confidently lean towards his sage advice. Many sources recommend taking the biofilm removing substance one half hour before you take anti-fungals.

Upon further research I learned another interesting tidbit: enzymes break down the cell walls of yeasts and candida. They also do this with little die-off symptoms and no resistance build-up issues. You should take a digestive enzyme supplement which contains protease, lipase, and amylase with every meal. The more easily digestible foods you eat—such as fish, steamed veggies, and no-sugar smoothies and green drinks—the more enzymes can go directly to work on the candida problem at hand.

In the chapter on enzymes and probiotics I explained how an ample supply of enzymes ensures health and vitality. If you are riddled with candida and eating the standard American diet, you are almost assuredly running a large deficit of much-needed enzymes and only aiding the candida to reproduce. Enzymes help to keep candida in check, but you must have enough left over after food digestion for them to work their magic.

Third Step: Anti-fungals

Anti-fungals need to be taken simultaneously with the anti-candida diet. There are prescription anti fungals like Amphotercin, Fluconazole (aka Diflucan), Itraconazole, Ketoconzaole, and Nystatin. These obviously require a doctor's prescription and are usually taken once a day. Botanical anti-fungals are: black walnut, garlic, uva ursi, wormwood, goldenseal, caprylic acid, oregano, olive leaf, cats claw, oil of thyme, and undecylenic acid. These can be taken 2 to 3 times daily. Botanical sources can be found easily at health food and vitamin stores. Some practitioners experienced with candida have suggested taking an anti-fungal for ten days and then rotating to a new one to avoid breeding resistance. This is when having a Susceptibility Profile is greatly helpful; you know to only rotate the anti-fungals that effectively destroy your personal invaders. If you are in doubt, try to find a health practitioner well acquainted with candidiasis to get a professional opinion on what to take, how much and when. Please note that anti-fungals should be taken on an empty stomach.

Fourth Step: Heal the Gut

In order to truly overcome candida, you must take probiotics to repopulate the intestines with healthy bacteria. These healthy bacteria keep biofilms from reoccurring and candida in check. Without probiotics to move into the space the candida have recently been evicted from, you are much more susceptible to another hostile takeover. As mentioned in a previous chapter, probiotics are the much needed back-up troops sent in to support your overworked immune army.

Look for a brand that provides at least 50-billion counts with as many strains as possible. Dan at www.yeastinfectionadvisor. com has researched the different brands on the market and how the strains work together. I suggest giving his free site a visit and doing some of your own research if you are unsure of what probiotic to buy.

Fifth Step: Keep Bowels Moving

If you are one of the many individuals who currently suffer or have ever suffered from constipation, you must clean out your colon. A stagnant colon quickly becomes putrid and becomes the perfect breeding ground for candida (not to mention parasites). In fact, by cleaning the colon you may notice a large portion of your problems disappear. If you have ever eaten a diet high in white flour, dairy, and sugar and low in fiber (which would be almost all Americans), you most likely have a cement-like toxic barrier built up along your colon walls. Diets high in processed dairy can also lead to mucosal build up along your intestines. Both of these substances need to exit the body so the colon can heal and get rid of toxins more effectively.

From extensive study of the benefits of a healthy large intestine, I found many sources that insist a clean colon is the key to great health.

While doing the candida cleanse, or perhaps up to 3 weeks beforehand, you want to increase your intake of fiber and natural substances that keep you moving. Vegetables have beneficial amounts of good fiber to aid this process. Probiotics taken daily also stimulate regular movements. Ground flaxseed and chia seed used in smoothies can also help greatly. If you have never done a colon detox, I found that the program and products at www. drnatura.com to be incredibly effective and did what they promised. Taking large amounts of magnesium or Epsom salts can cure small bouts of constipation but does not necessarily remove plaque or build-up in the colon.

If you have suffered for many years with constipation, I would recommend a colon detox cleanse first. This gives your body the raw materials it needs to clean its own house. If the colon detox does not finish the job, professional colonics may be required.

Trying to rid yourself of candida with a toxic colon is counter-productive. You need all channels open to get rid of the toxins and die-off that results from the first four steps of the cleanse.

Super Bonus Idea: Having A Clean Liver

Just like the colon, if the liver is backed-up with toxins and parasites, it cannot assist you in clearing out candida. In fact, a toxic liver may be one of the causes of candida overpopulation in the first place. While researching possible causes of illness and depression I stumbled upon a liver cleanse protocol that I now jokingly call: The Liver Blow. The name is a joke, but the effects are not. I have done this cleanse multiple times and am amazed by the results. Overall, I give this cleanse 2 thumbs up but you must be prepared! If you do not first get your body ready for this cleanse you could have a terrible experience.

The premise behind the cleanse is that the liver and gall-bladder ducts get blocked from time to time with toxic sludge or stones that need to be assisted out of the body. If you have ever had a gallstone causing a gallbladder attack, you know this can be happen quite unexpectedly and be excruciatingly painful. Parasites can also block liver pathways and wreak havoc on this already overworked organ. These blockages and toxic sludge are believed to be the source of allergies, fatigue, and lack of sense of well-being.

A clean liver is undoubtedly a desirable asset. But if you are getting rid of candida, it becomes even more important. All the toxins of candida die-off must be removed through the liver. Depending on how much overgrowth you have, this can be a huge job. In order to minimize the misery, you would be wise to make sure your liver is clean and able to handle the load.

I have read hundreds of personal testimonies about the miraculous turn-around in people's health after doing a liver cleanse (or in many cases, a series of liver cleanses). I have also read many personal stories of horrible experiences and doctors who disdain this cleanse as "ridiculous and unhelpful." As mentioned before, I've done it myself many times. I found a renewed energy and sense of well-being. I also noticed the whites of my eyes became whiter. But one time I had a terrible experience because I had not prepared correctly. I had not done a parasite cleanse or stayed current on parasite prevention supplements. I had also not eaten apples or taken apple cider vinegar the week before which can soften stones in the liver and gallbladder. As a result, I was nauseas for hours and eventually vomited during the night of the cleanse. It was the least fun thing I can imagine doing to oneself on purpose. Don't make that mistake!

Now that you have been warned, the cleanse works like this:

1. Make sure you are free of parasites by doing a parasite cleanse or remaining on parasite prevention protocol. (View Dr. Clark's parasite cleanse at www.drclark.net for an excellent, natural protocol. You can also purchase the ingredients at www.drclarkstore.com.)
2. Plan a day where you can do the cleanse when you have the following day to recover.
3. For the 5 days leading up to the cleanse, eat at least an apple a day and try to get 1 Tbsp of raw apple cider vinegar per day (more is fine too).

4. On the day of the cleanse eat only foods with no fats or proteins such as oatmeal, fruit, rice, and plain vegetables up until 2 pm. This allows bile to build up in the gallbladder. Do not eat anything after 2 pm.

5. At 6 pm take the equivalent of 1 tablespoon of Epsom salts dissolved in 16 ounces of water (it tastes awful—you have been warned!) or take the equivalent of 1 Tbsp of Epsom salt in capsules and drink 2 cups of water. The magnesium in Epsom salts relaxes the bile ducts of the liver and gallbladder as well as the sphincters within the small and large intestines. Expect diarrhea as your body empties the colon.

6. At 8 pm take one more dose of Epsom salts to drive that message of relaxation all the way home. You will be going to the bathroom a lot.

7. At 9:45 make sure you are almost ready to go to bed. Hit the bathroom one last time. At 10 pm mix ½ cup of light-tasting olive oil and ½ cup of freshly squeezed (by you, just moments earlier) room-temp grapefruit juice in a shaker cup. Mix vigorously and it won't taste so bad. I use a straw to then suck this concoction down as quickly as possible. Take less than 10 minutes to do this, as you need to get into bed and try to sleep quickly. Make sure your bed is ready and that you can be uninterrupted during the night (your spouse needs to take on kid-duty if necessary). The fat in this mixture triggers the gallbladder and liver to release bile at a rapid rate. As your ducts are now relaxed, stones and other sludge are pushed down through the system and into the colon. Some experts say to sleep on your right side, but it makes me feel sick so I sleep on my back with my torso and head slightly elevated.

8. The next morning (meaning any time after 6 am), take

another 1 Tbsp dose of Epsom salts with lots of water and lie down.

9. Two hours later, take your last 1 Tbsp dose of Epsom salts. Throughout the morning you will pass greenish stones though the colon. Some may be very large, some will be tiny. Every single stone exiting the body is a good thing. These stones will float as they are largely made up of bile and cholesterol. There is controversy on whether these stones were blocking the liver or were made during the night after the large intake of olive oil. I know I have passed stones so large there is no way they were made overnight. I am a believer in this cleanse.

10. You can drink juices two hours later but start whole food slowly. Dr. Clark recommends juice first, then fruit twenty minutes later, then food an hour after that.

I tweaked this protocol by merging the best ideas from several different sources and my own experiences. However, many people cite the originator of this protocol to be Hulda Regehr Clark. All of Dr. Clark's recipes can be found readily on the internet. She was a great believer in people having access to inexpensive methods of healing themselves and many today swear that her insights healed them from cancer, infertility, and more.

Liver cleansing can be done every two weeks if you feel up to it. Others space out their cleansing 4 to 6 weeks apart. The goal is to get around 2000 stones removed before you can count on large improvements in health.

What Next?

After you have completed 2 to 4 weeks on the strict anti-candida diet, you may try introducing fruits. Watch for signs of candida repopulation such as brain fog, lack of well-being, or fatigue. If fruits do not jive with you just yet you may need to continue on the strict portion of the diet. Try again in another week.

The goal is to eventually get to the point where fruits, grains, and starchy vegetables eaten in moderation do not cause a major setback. But you will never again be allowed to eat white flour, sugar, and processed grains as part of your daily diet. The truth is, after removing candida from your system you will not crave or desire junk. Your only job now is to not allow it to creep back into your life. A candida relapse is no picnic. And now that you know how the die-off portion works, you probably have no desire to go there again. Think of your new lifestyle as a mandatory healthy diet. Your health and happiness depends on it.

The good news is that there are many Paleo cookbooks that are great for the maintenance portion of the candida diet. The Paleo diet is becoming more and more popular because it resolves many people's health issues. I'm not surprised—the Paleo diet naturally weakens candida and starves it at the source. The Paleo diet also eliminates most foods that have been altered in a lab like wheat, corn, and soy. Is it any wonder that this diet makes people feel better?

If you need help with recipe ideas, I highly recommend visiting Paleo websites for a quick hit of inspiration. Remember: it might be hard, but getting rid of candida is absolutely worth doing. Take control of your life and get your health back!

Chapter 14

TO FAST OR NOT TO FAST:

The Key to Restoring Your Health

Fasting has been part of human culture since the beginning of recorded history. The technical definition of fasting is to willingly abstain from some or all food and drink for a period of time. The key word there is *willingly*. Fasting is a choice—not an affliction.

Most religions have some form of fasting in their cultural traditions. The Bible records that Moses, King David, and Jesus all fasted for spiritual guidance. Muslims fast during the daylight hours throughout the 40 days of Ramadan. Jews fast on Yom Kippur and Tisha B'Av, among other days. Buddhist monks and nuns are known to practice intermittent fasting. And Eastern Orthodox Christians have four different fasting seasons, including two stretches of 40 days. There are many other sects and religions that have some aspect of fasting in their traditions as well.

In my church, we are asked to fast from all food and drink on the first Sunday of each month. Church members usually start their fast after dinner on Saturday night and end it on Sunday evening. We also have a tradition of fasting and praying whenever we need additional support through difficult trials.

With all this talk of religion and fasting you might think that the two necessarily go together. But that is not the case. Fasting is a tool available to anyone. And if you eat the Standard American Diet, you might want to consider taking advantage of it more often. In this chapter I will explain the benefits of fasting, how it can help you recover your vitality, and why it is the health cure that no one talks about.

Benefits of Fasting

Dozens of studies show that fasting has many beneficial effects on the human body. Contrary to what the food industry has told us, humans can tolerate a lot of missed meals. Doing so can help you recover from cravings, food intolerances, and raised insulin levels just to name a few. Furthermore, cognitive awareness, memory, and energy levels can soar in as little as 16 hours of fasting.

Documented benefits of fasting include:

- Decreased insulin levels, which allow your body to stop storing energy as fat
- Decreased blood glucose levels, which allows stored fat to be used for fuel
- Increased mental clarity
- Increased levels of BDNF, a protein that protects the brain against age-related mental decline and is necessary for learning
- Increased growth hormone levels which burn fat and increase metabolism
- Increased epinephrine and norepinephrine levels which increase energy and alertness

- Lean muscle mass retention despite fears of muscle atrophy from fasting
- Fat and weight loss with no other dietary restrictions after the fast has ended

The magic time range for getting the most from your fast is 18 to 24 hours. At that point, blood glucose levels have dramatically decreased and many of the health benefits have been reached[43]. Upon waking in the morning, if you were to simply avoid food until 1 or 2 pm you could complete a 16 hour fast with little to no effort. You can fast two separate days a week if you are healthy.

Fasting for the first time can be challenging. Your body is used to three meals a day—plus snacks. If you eat a lot of processed flour and sugar, fasting will be tough. However, if you eat a healthy diet with little sugar, fasting will be much less painful. Either way, fasting gets easier the more you do it. You will notice less bodily resistance each time you deprive yourself of food. Our bodies were made for intermittent fasting—they thrive on it.

Regardless of what experts and scientific studies say, breakfast is not the most important meal of the day—nor is lunch, or dinner for that matter. Your body can handle long stretches without food. The main exceptions to this rule are if you are diabetic, pregnant, or nursing. You should never fast under those conditions unless you clear it with your doctor first. Furthermore, if you suffer from adrenal fatigue as explained in Chapter 17, fasting is not your friend. Eat small, frequent meals, heal your adrenals, and then consider fasting.

If you are fasting for religious reasons and the guidelines exclude drinking liquids, follow your heart. But on days that you fast for your health alone, I suggest drinking lots of water to help eliminate unwanted toxins. As discussed in the chapter on enzymes and probiotics, when your give your body a break from digestion your enzyme factories shift from digestion to metabolization. This means your enzyme cleaning crews start working overtime on repair and garbage removal. Without water, the job of removing these unwanted substances is significantly tougher and you may start to feel sick.

Another benefit of fasting was discovered by accident. I personally found that during a time of hyper-sensitivity to foods, when my body seemed to react to almost everything I ate, that fasting seemed to reset both my intestines and my immune system. If you ever find yourself afraid of food, try a 24 hour fast. You may find that it is the magic reset button you've been looking for.

Why You've Never Heard of Fasting to Regain Your Health

The real reason no doctor, pharmaceutical company, food manufacturer or supplement distributor will tell you fasting can heal your body is because of one thing: money. They don't make any revenue if you heal yourself. Why would they try to make themselves or their products obsolete? The real truth is that it takes **nothing** to yield the greatest results in regaining your health. No food, no snacks, no powdered drinks, no pills—literally nothing.

Fasting helps the body catch up on all its back-logged tasks—just as an extra day off work allows you to catch up on bills, taxes, mail, and all those other things you've been meaning to do. Fasting allows the gut to heal and take a well-deserved rest. Fasting is the key to maintaining good health and vitality.

If you thought fasting was just a spiritual test—I invite you to now reconsider. Fasting in these days is almost crucial to giving your body a much-needed break. In fact, we would do well to consider fasting on a weekly basis. Consider it a gift to your body, mind, and spirit. It might be the best gift you ever give yourself.

Chapter 15
HORMONES AND INFERTILITY:
The Bane of Female Existence

I would surmise that every woman has dealt with a hormonal melt down at least once in her life. The feeling of being overwhelmed, angry, and offended all at once is not unusual for women. Nor is feeling incredibly sad and broken. The kicker is that our emotions are often stronger and more confusing than we realize because of the delicate dance known as hormonal balance.

I like to think that women in times past had an easier time of it. I like to think that they had easy, breezy monthly cycles and that pregnancies came easily to them. I think for the most part, that was probably true. But even historically women had problems with fertility, as noted in the Bible several times. Some individuals' fertility and hormone problems cannot be fixed, are known by God, and are part of His plan. But just in case they are reversible, here's what you need to know.

Every hormone is created from cholesterol. Yes, CHOLESTEROL—the same substance that doctors give people statins to keep at lower levels. New research is emerging that is blowing the whistle on the widely held medical belief that cholesterol is bad for you and causes heart problems[44]. Cholesterol is a powerful antioxidant that helps restore inflamed tissues. It also protects the brain from dementia, Parkinson's, and Alzheimer's[45]. Studies have shown that individuals with higher cholesterol levels have a lower risk of diabetes and dementia in their later years[46]. In the case of excessively high cholesterol levels, as mentioned in the chapter on fats, reducing inflammation in the body naturally balances cholesterol levels. This is best accomplished by eliminating genetically modified grains, pasteurized dairy, and sugar. Most of what you may have been taught on cholesterol is wrong—and I wonder whose plan it was to confuse the masses?

Your body can make cholesterol in the liver. But if you consume it through food, your liver will cut back on its own production. Eggs, butter, and shellfish are high cholesterol foods that have been vilified over the last several decades. Interestingly, eggs, butter, and seafood keep popping up on my research radar as foods that support fertility, brain health, and decent hormonal function. Do not be afraid of these foods. Ignore all the noise and listen for the signal of truth. These foods have supported life for millennia. Our ancestors ate them on a regular basis. They are full of nutrients that our bodies crave. Just make sure they come from clean, wild, and properly fed and cared-for sources.

Hormone production also requires Vitamin A for every conversion: from cholesterol to pregnenalone to progesterone, estradiol, and testosterone. As discussed in an earlier chapter, we are not giving our bodies the vital, easily useable Vitamin A from organ meats, cod liver oil, and raw, full-fat dairy products that our ancestors consumed for healthy hormone production. These food sources also provide essential fats and minerals necessary for hormonal creation and removal.

Calcium and magnesium are especially crucial to our monthly cycles and to maintaining some level of emotional stability during the monthly rollercoaster rides. Calcium deficiency has been hyped in recent years, and most women try to get increased amounts. But magnesium is noticeably deficient in our current diets. As mentioned in an earlier chapter, magnesium is required for over 300 enzymatic functions. With low levels, our monthly cycles and fertility are negatively impacted.

High stress levels inhibit healthy hormone production. Constant stress robs your body of Vitamin A when the adrenals deem the stress response to be a higher priority than fertility or stable moods. This happens when Vitamin A and cholesterol are "robbed" from their intended purpose of creating sex hormones and are instead used to make cortisol, the stress-managing hormone. The constant stress women deal with today is taxing our entire hormonal cascade and making us temperamental, overwhelmed, and infertile in the process. We must realize that external stress is mostly a "perceived" threat. Meaning that we create our own stress by how we allow events and situations to affect us. Stress is so pervasive that it gets its own chapter where we will discuss strategies on how to combat this current-day epidemic.

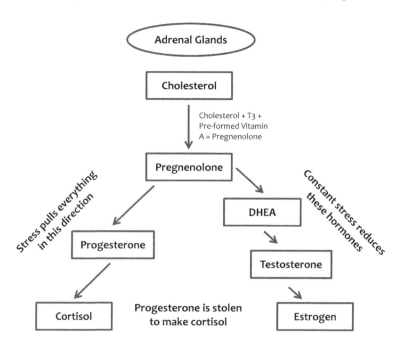

Once sex hormones are created, they are picked up by receptor sites throughout the body. When everything is working properly, these sites pick up the roving hormones, utilize them appropriately and then discard them. Unfortunately there are two problems that can occur here:

1. clogged receptor sites, and
2. poor breakdown of used hormones.

BHT, phthalates, and other preservatives and chemicals in our food and beauty products disrupt hormonal function when they jump on our receptor sites and refuse to get off. Like a bully who won't give other kids a turn at the merry-go-round, these substances block the receptor sites from being used the way they were intended. The sites are full and simply cannot pick up the needed hormones for our bodies to use. Avoid personal products and plastic goods that have these chemicals. These hormone-disrupting substances are banned in other countries. Why they are still legal in the United States is a mystery. They are not friends to your monthly cycles or your fertility.

Other things that can clog your receptor sites are genetically modified foods such as soy. It is no secret that soy has been scientifically altered from its natural state. Genetic modifications have allowed more soy to be grown around the world and more soy products to enter the market. It is likely that you eat several things each day containing soy ingredients without even knowing it. Soy production is big business. But even before genetic modifications existed, ancient Asians documented that soy had enzyme inhibitors that wreak havoc on the intestines, block mineral absorption, and cause internal stress. Soy is also a known estrogen impersonator. The presence of it in your body sends signals that you have plenty of estrogen and no more is required. Like the game of telephone, where the initial message gets massacred as it is whispered down the line, the message received at the final destination is incorrect. If you have hormonal issues, please avoid soy.

Candida, an invasive form of yeast in the human body, can block hormone receptor sites as well. It is very likely the hidden source of many women's hormonal issues. Our poor diets and the exposure to more and more toxins can alter the pH balance in the intestines. This imbalance is unfavorable to our good bacteria but very favorable to the growth of candida. See Chapter 13 for detailed information on how candida occurs and how to evict this unwanted occupant.

The second issue mentioned above, poor breakdown of used hormones, is another problem that may need attention. Some women have a genetic weakness in breaking down and discarding these used hormones. If you decide to get a genetic test run from Genovations (as mentioned in Chapter 12 on toxicity), make sure to check your COMT gene which regulates the breakdown of estrogen. Any anomaly on this gene pair could mean your body needs extra assistance as explained below. I have an anomaly in this area and if you have hormone issues, you may as well. (I hypothesize that my pregnancies were exceptionally difficult because of my malnourished state and genetic weakness at breaking down estrogen—which is created in large quantities while pregnant.)

Once the hormone has served its purpose on the receptor site it needs to be broken down to be excreted into our trash removal system. This conversion is supposed to be quick and effortless. However, if the conversion isn't performed properly you can end up with dangerous substances hanging around in the body. To get rid of these substances, you need large amounts of cruciferous vegetables and trace minerals.

Supplementation with bioavailable Diindolylmethane (the

substance found in broccoli, cauliflower, and cabbage), also known as DIM, is another way to assist your body in this removal process. In addition, I have found drinking a mixture of 1 scoop of VegeSplash (Super ORAC Concentrated Greens Drink Mix—apple and carrot flavor) in 8 ounces of water each day is an easy way to get the needed substances and helps me to feel significantly better. It is a powerhouse of good veggies and greens: broccoli, beets, celery, kale, carrots, onions, kombu seaweed, wakame seaweed, nori seaweed, Hawaiian blue-green algae and added enzymes. You can find it on Amazon.com. I have taken this product for years and notice that I have better moods and overall health when consuming it. The extra bonus of added digestive enzymes helps to take stress off the pancreas and allow it to create more metabolic enzymes as well.

Once you get your hormone receptor sites cleaned and cleared, and dispose of unwanted hormonal by-products, you could notice a significant change in your overall moods and vitality. But this change can only occur when the body has all the raw materials it needs to make hormones in the first place.

In order to provide your body these raw materials you must have a healthy diet and a healthy gut. Circling back to the chapter on your brain and the gut, a healthy brain *requires* a healthy gut. Healthy hormones require the same. If your gut is inflamed, irritated, or fighting against gluten or other food intolerances, your body will be in a constant state of stress. That is in addition to all the other outside stressors you deal with every day. If your immune system residing in the gut is going haywire, your non-essential hormones (such as reproductive and mood-balancing hormones) will come in dead last on the priority scale. Your adrenals will become fatigued from fighting constant inflammation and not be able to create the range of hormones necessary for fertility and balanced monthly cycles.

Additionally, an inflamed gut doesn't allow for proper absorption of vital nutrients necessary for hormones to be created. It is a catch-22, no-win situation. You could be eating what you consider to be an amazingly healthy diet but nothing is getting to the right place. I did this for years, and I'm telling you that keeping pizza and doughnuts in your diet if they are decimating your intestines—even when combined with all kinds of other healthier foods—is *not* worth it.

If you are sensitive to the common offenders like gluten or dairy, it may have started with one too many rounds of antibiotics or a highly stressful time in your life. The good bacteria in your gut were depleted and your immune system went a little haywire. If you catch it fast enough and do a gut repair job with probiotics and easily digestible food, you can possibly reset your immune system and enjoy most foods again. If, however, you knowingly or unknowingly keep plodding on for years eating things your body has decided it needs to fight, you may end up with a stubborn immune system that begins to react to almost every food you eat. After that, hormonal imbalance is simply the confirmation of years of inflammation and stress on your body.

You may need bio-identical hormones to assist the body in healing from years of stress and disrepair. If you have issues sleeping, you are bound to have several crucial parts of your health disrupted, including your hormone production. The problem is yet another catch-22; you need hormones to sleep properly so your body can mend and make more hormones. If you are absolutely unable to regulate your sleep patterns, you will probably need hormonal help.

The Adversary did a great job scaring women away from hormone assistance with the recent turmoil of information over hormone replacement therapy (HRT). It all started with pharmaceutical companies creating their own formulas that they could then patent. You see, it is illegal to patent substances found organically in nature, and therefore, pharmaceutical companies cannot make large quantities of money from something already existing in our biological environment. They had to alter it, package it, and market it as something that would help women suffering from hormonal imbalance and its effects. The problem occurred when their formulas of altered hormones caused increased incidents of heart disease and other health issues and the whistle was blown.

Be assured that the formulas pharmaceutical companies make are NOT found naturally in nature. However, bio-identical hormones are *biologically identical* to the ones your body makes and can be a great tool for regaining your health.

The confusion the Adversary caused was just enough to make the average woman doubt the efficacy and safety of bio-identical hormones. Just enough doubt and fear will keep good people from doing great things. When considering taking bio-identical hormones, the hope is that you will not need them forever, but can use them as a way to re-start your body's own natural hormonal processes. To stay on the safe side, you probably want to use them only as long as absolutely necessary. Ask friends for referrals or check online for a qualified doctor who can become familiar with your issues and prescribe these for you.

Lessons In Illness and Infertility

From 1932 to 1942, Dr. Frances Pottenger ran an experiment to determine the effect of heat-processed food on cats. Over a period of ten years, he documented and studied the results of five groups of cats over four generations. Two groups were fed raw milk, cod liver oil and raw beef liver, heart, brain, and muscle scraps (note that this was before cows were fed genetically modified corn) while the other three groups were fed a diet of cooked meat and pasteurized, evaporated, and condensed milk.

The first generation of all three groups fed processed milk and cooked meat developed diseases and illnesses near the end of their lives. The second generation of the three groups fed this same diet developed diseases and illnesses in the middle of their lives. The third generation fed this diet developed diseases and illnesses in the beginning of their lives and many died before six months of age. There was no fourth generation in any of the three processed milk and cooked meat food groups. Either the third generation parents were sterile or the fourth generation cats died before birth.

All four generations of groups fed raw meat and raw milk remained healthy throughout their normal lifespans and had no fertility problems.

As for applying his results to human nutrition, Dr. Pottenger said, "While no attempt will be made to correlate the changes in the animals studied with malformations found in humans, the similarity is so obvious that parallel pictures will suggest themselves."

If you are eating the Standard American Diet, the only question is: Which malnourished generation are you in?

Restoring Fertility

As mentioned previously, infertility is a trial that some couples are not meant to overcome. Some children are destined to arrive at their intended family through adoption. But in case you have a situation that can be corrected, here are some natural protocols that work. Just note that both you and your spouse need to follow these guidelines. This is not a one-person task.

1. Change your diet.
   a. Omit wheat, conventional dairy, corn, and soy—anything that has been genetically modified—as well as any food with preservatives, "natural" flavors, artificial flavors, and/or man-made colorings and chemicals.
   b. Eat only organic produce and grains and up your intake of fruits and vegetables.
   c. Make sure the proteins you eat are organic or humanely raised and fed including beef, poultry, eggs, pork, and bison. Ensure any fish you eat is not farmed, and avoid high-mercury fish like tuna, orange roughy, mackerel, shark, and swordfish.
   d. Eat organic beef and chicken livers once to twice a week. The vitamin and mineral content in these organ meats is nutritionally unparalleled.
   e. Eat only healthy fats and plenty of them—olive oil, pastured, grass-fed butter and cream (especially from cows eating growing spring grasses), coconut oil, avocados, cod liver oil. Absolutely no "vegetable" oil, soybean oil, cottonseed oil, canola oil, or rapeseed oil unless they are organic and even then only in very small quantities.
   f. Drink a green drink everyday with enzymes (either freshly juiced or as a lesser option, VegeSplash mentioned earlier in this chapter).
   g. Eat properly fermented foods to aid digestion like sauerkraut, kimchi, raw milk yogurt, and beet kvass.
   h. Add clean seafoods to your diet that are rich in trace minerals and healthy fats like sardines, oysters, mussels, and fish eggs.
   i. Eliminate all sugar. You can use honey or stevia only. Absolutely NO diet sodas.

Basically, eat like you lived 500 years ago. Yes, it may sound expensive—but it is far cheaper than even one round of in-vitro fertilization.

2. Exercise 3-5 days a week for at least 30 minutes. Make sure to sweat in order to eliminate toxins held in your body's tissues.
3. Drink lots of filtered water to carry away toxins and make sure your cells are properly hydrated.
4. Take digestive enzymes with meals and probiotics daily to support nutrient absorption.
5. Change your health care products as advised in Chapter 12 on toxicity.
6. Take no pharmaceuticals or over-the-counter medications unless absolutely necessary.
7. Take high-quality vitamin supplements that include vitamins A, D, E, K and C and all the B vitamins along with the trace minerals like selenium, zinc, iodine, copper, and chromium. You may need to take iron separately. These supplements are an insurance plan so that every organ and cell you have has access to the nutrients it needs. And don't forget to supplement the major minerals like magnesium and calcium!
8. Relax. You must stop the cycle of stress-induced cortisol-production robbing the precursors needed for your fertility hormones. Do yoga, go on a vacation with lots of sun and water, and/or change careers. Do whatever you have to do to reduce or eliminate stress in your life. This is an absolute necessity.
9. Sleep. You must get at least 7 to 8 hours of sleep a night for your organs to rest and reset your hormone levels.

I have many friends who have children because of the assistance of fertility doctors and pharmaceuticals. If you can afford it, I wish you all the best. But before you shell out tens of thousands of dollars, try the above suggestions for 6 months. You may be able to avoid debt or put that money into your child's education fund instead.

In Summary

The best way to balance your hormones and regain your vitality, moods, and fertility is to fix your gut, avoid food allergens, decrease your internal and external stressors, eat and use clean foods and personal products, eat only good fats, and provide your body with foods that are nutrient dense. Supplement your diet with high-quality vitamins, Vitamin D, magnesium and calcium, and fermented cod liver oil from reputable sources (contains easily assimilated Vitamin A).

By the word "clean" I mean non-genetically modified foods and products free of man-made chemicals and pesticides. Nutrient dense foods are organ meats, pastured animal proteins fed a clean diet, wild-caught cold-water fish, cod liver oil, coconut oil, butter, olive oil, fermented foods, and organic fruits and vegetables straight from the ground. Make your own condiments and salad dressings and cook at home. Furthermore, you may want to get a diagnosis of your genetics from Genova Diagnostics (www.gdx. net) to see if you need additional hormonal clearing support. If necessary, don't be afraid to seek bio-identical hormone assistance to regain your good health.

The best way to keep your hormones and fertility imbalanced and erratic is to eat lots of sugar, wheat, genetically modified soy and corn, pasteurized milk and cheese products, caffeine, rancid and processed fats, never take vitamins or probiotics, use loads of chemical-laden personal products, and experience lots of stress.

If it is at all possible to regain hormonal balance and fertility, you now know how to turn it around. It may not seem easy, but the power is in you—and your health and happiness are worth it. From one sister who's been there to another, I send you hope for a more sane and stable future!

Chapter 16
STRESS:

An Unforgiving Master

Our world today is full of stress. Whether you are married, single, with or without children, your day is full of things you need and want to do. Relationships, too little or too much exercise, traffic, personal goals, work deadlines, meal preparation—all happen every day. Some things we must do and others we *think* we must do in order to be successful, healthy, or accepted by society and our peers.

In The American Psychological Association's 2012 annual survey on stress, women reported higher levels of stress than men as well as increased feelings of inadequacy in that they are not handling their stresses well. Another interesting factor in the study was the analysis of caregivers—a job which commonly falls to women. Not surprisingly, caregivers reported the highest levels of stress with little to no time for themselves in which to recover.

Whether we like it or not, women carry the lion's share of responsibility in the care and feeding of their families—both immediate and extended. Add in a job, volunteer work, church responsibilities, and exercise regime, and you've already over-scheduled yourself. All of the things we try to do chip away at our energy stores and reserves. If we accidentally hit our physical limit and can no longer function, the world as we know it could begin to crumble. Spouses and children suffer, employers are left in the lurch, volunteer work goes undone, and bank accounts become overdrawn when women can't accomplish all the things required of them.

In this chapter we will discuss how you can protect yourself from ever-increasing amounts of stress. But first, another cautionary tale.

A Little Story About Stress

On January 1st during my senior year of high school, my parents told my sister and me that they were getting a divorce. I was shocked. My parents never fought. I'd rarely even seen them have a disagreement of any kind, but suddenly here they were getting a divorce.

They went to counseling, but it was too late. Their neglected marriage was beyond repair. As the years passed, I began to grasp why it had happened. But that understanding only came with a lot of time. That January morning I could not understand how two people who had been together over 25 years could simply stop loving each other. I began to believe marriage was a sham and that love was a joke.

My brother was on a two-year mission to Germany at the time—just 4 months out. We decided the work he was doing was more important than anything going on at home and that he deserved to do it without any unnecessary distractions. There was no rush to finalize matters, so we agreed to keep this news from him and our other relatives. My sister and I only told one trustworthy friend apiece, and that was it. No extended family, no other friends. We sat on our sad secret and wondered what it meant for the future.

For me, my friends took the place of my family. As soon as I realized my family wasn't going to be a cohesive unit, I felt disjointed and disconnected. I felt like I had a mother, a father, a brother, and a sister individually—but I did not have a family.

What I did have was a very close group of friends who hung out all the time. We had big dreams of graduating from college and taking on the world. We supported each other in studying, achieving and playing hard. These friends took the place of my family. They set a high standard for what a friend was supposed to be—supportive and honest. Not telling most of my friends about the divorce felt deceitful and underhanded. It became more and more taxing as time went on.

Going off to Provo, Utah, that fall was even more challenging. Having never been west of the Mississippi River, Utah was a bit of a shock to my system. I knew very few people and had no close friends at BYU. I had to start over completely. I was severely homesick and friend-sick, but I also felt that I was where I needed to be. My body decided that all the new difficulties of college classes, tons of homework, no family and no close friends was a bit too much. My face started breaking out and I had trouble sleeping.

I described how during my sophomore year at BYU I almost changed schools because of severe depression in the chapter titled "In The Beginning," so I won't cover that again. But it was an extremely stressful time. I repented for my poor choices and made necessary changes. But I had to speak with a Stake President in order to stay at BYU. He just happened to be George D. Durrant, a well-known LDS author, speaker, and educator. During our discussion, I could feel his love and concern. I explained how if I had

had a close friend there it would have made a huge difference. His closing words to me were, "A friend, huh?"

That summer I went to Alaska with my best friend from Alabama who had been attending Ricks College. Her roommate knew other students who had worked at fish canneries in Alaska. She got us applications which we promptly sent in. We were elated to receive job offers and went two summers in a row. It was an amazing learning experience and each summer we came home with a huge paycheck. But we also worked 16 to 20 hour days for weeks on end. I didn't realize it at the time because I was 19 and thought I was invincible, but working long hours and going without sleep is hard on the body. It was a stressor that I underestimated.

Four months after speaking with George D. Durrant I returned to BYU and met someone who became, and is still, one of my best friends to this day. Her name happens to be Charity (God has a sense of humor, so help me). She had started her own company in her teens and was a professional working woman by 20. She opened my eyes to what life could offer and I began to paint a bigger picture for my future. She also introduced me to a plethora of new friends and people who I connected with instantly. I felt a wave of relief wash over me—I *can* fit in here. There are people here like me. But it did not go unnoticed that none of these blessings occurred until after I humbled my heart towards God, exercised faith and took the harder path. In hindsight, the choice to remain at BYU was the best I could have made. But because of my ignorance about depression, the entire experience still caused lots of stress, both physical and mental.

The next January, I got the privilege of attending the London BYU study abroad program. Our group studied British history there, as well as British literature and fine art. The topics we studied were the polar opposite of those required by someone majoring in economics, and I treasured the knowledge from that experience. Unfortunately, it came with an unanticipated and heavy cost. At the end of the semester that April, I returned to Alabama for the summer in bad shape. After spending the winter in a cloudy, overcast city I experienced more depression that I ever had before. Perhaps it was a lack of good nutrition, mercury toxicity released from burning coal, or the toxins from the brake dust in the Tube (the London subway), but I was beyond low. This was a scary kind of depression—the kind that makes you not want to wake up in the morning—and I had no idea at the time what was wrong with me.

I decided to cut my summer time in Alabama short and head back to Utah to try and recover among friends. After two months of lying out in the Utah sun, sleeping, working an easy job and reconnecting with people, I started to be able to see light at the end of the depression tunnel (Vitamin D is a powerful hormone—make no mistake!). It was a good thing, too, because fall semester of my senior year at BYU required every ounce of energy I had. I was taking the hardest classes for my major, studying for the GRE (Graduate Record Exam—necessary to apply to many graduate schools), applying and interviewing for jobs, running weekly church social events for a group of 150 students, setting up recruiting events for the Economics club, and still managing to have a social life. It was the busiest, most exhilarating time of my life and with a lot of prayer and daily planning I was blessed to fit everything in.

I never entertained the thought of dating seriously or getting married while at BYU because of my parents' divorce. I did not believe love could last. What was the point if you just fell out of love 25 years later? I had no desire to even try. I focused on getting a good job and going to graduate school. I hung out with the other motivated guys in my major (because it was 99% male), and we swapped recruiting information and interview prep questions. Looking back, I'm grateful for the experience but realize how the Adversary played on my disbelief in marriage to keep me isolated and stand-offish. I was not "flirty" or open to being asked out. I had lots of guy friends but only went out on one official date the entire time I attended BYU.

The next summer I started a job in San Francisco in the high-tech consulting industry. Starting over again was stressful, but not as hard as BYU had been. Around this time, I started to take a long-term round of antibiotics prescribed by my dermatologist to clear up my skin. I was tired of dealing with breakouts and this direction was what the doctor suggested. I didn't know then that those antibiotics would decimate the probiotic balance in my intestines and cause years of future suffering.

I had also unwisely accumulated debt during my senior year of college thinking I was going to have a great job and pay it off easily. It was a hard, cold realization when I learned that San Francisco rents and entry-level paychecks did not get along well. I had to pinch pennies to pay down that debt every month, and it still took 3 years. I learned that debt is a heavy burden to bear—and not worth any short-term buying thrill. Coincidentally, I began to experience extreme shoulder and neck tension. Being 22, I just contributed it to working at a computer all day and ignored it.

The constant travel I had to do for my job was another challenge. The company would fly us home for weekends, but it was difficult to date or volunteer in the community when evenings were usually spent in another city. I was an uber-deluxe frequent-flyer by the age of 23. Most of the flight attendants didn't believe me when I tried to board with the men during the call for frequent flyers. I had to keep proof at the ready. Living out of a suitcase and vying with other travelers each week for luggage space, rental cars, and hotel shuttles with my neck and back muscles in knots was not fun. And it was definitely stressful.

Realizing you hate your job is stressful. Having a limited support system and longing to live closer to family is stressful. Finally letting go and falling in love with someone only to have your heart broken is stressful. But quitting your job, moving to another state and recovering from a breakup at the same time is apparently not a good idea. When you fill up your stress bucket to the brim, it doesn't take much for it to get maxed out and overflow.

And it wasn't just moving and starting a new job that was stressful—my health was starting to show signs of wear and tear. I had extreme muscle tension consistently and headaches to go along with it. My energy was waning and so was my focus at work. Depression was starting to rear its ugly head again. I forced myself through each day with it nipping at my heels.

It's funny how people make the same mistakes over and over again. Leave one high-tech job because you hate it, then get another that looks just like it (but says it won't make you travel as much—they promise!) In the dot-com era, it was commonplace for people to work themselves to the bone for stock options. We were all going to be millionaires! It's okay to run on adrenaline—you're young, right? But being in charge of over-sold, under-staffed projects is beyond stressful—it becomes downright painful. Next you might be told to go save a project in another state that is on the brink of ruin which leads to more travel, more stress, more headaches. No dating, no family or friends to rely on—just you and the mortgage you need to pay. A mortgage for a place you only visit on weekends.

You know you need to quit this job but you have no time to look when you work 6 days a week for 14 hours straight. Not to mention you're in a different city from where you live so it's hard to make it to an interview.

All it takes at this point is one surgery, one hard recovery, and one last round of antibiotics for stress to put the final nail in the coffin. And all you can do is watch as your health drains away for good.

Lessons Learned

If you've pushed your body past the breaking point before you even consider having children, you put yourself In a precarious position. Pregnancy and raising toddlers is one of the hardest jobs on the planet and requires every ounce of energy you have. It most definitely tops the High Stress Jobs list. You need to make sure to leave some reserves for the task of raising a family or you may find you have nothing left for the most important people in your life.

From the above experiences I learned that emotional, physical, and mental stress all drain the body's resources—regardless of their origin. But while some stressors are out of our control, others are entirely within our realm of influence. There are important steps we can take to handle, redirect, or remove the pressures of daily life—we just need to know what they are and how to apply them. With this knowledge, I hope you can learn how to protect yourself from many of the causes of health-deteriorating, unrelenting stress.

The main thing you must understand is that stress triggers your body to make **cortisol**. This substance slows digestion, releases excess glucose into the blood stream, and increases the appetite for quick energy (like sugar and carbs)—all of which promote weight gain. Elevated cortisol levels for extended periods of time can disturb sleep cycles and promote moodiness, memory loss, and brain fog. Furthermore the production of cortisol requires Vitamin A and pregnenalone which is the precursor to progesterone. If you are experiencing frequent stress, your body will curtail its production of progesterone to account for increasing demands for cortisol which can lead to decreased libido and fertility problems.

A secondary issue caused by stress occurs when the pituitary gland stimulates the thyroid to produce thyroxine. Thyroxine causes a boost in heart rate, blood-sugar levels, blood pressure, and respiration so you can quickly run from an attacker. Unfortunately, increased thyroxine levels also cause the body to pull deeply from its nutrient stores. This metabolic boost burns through B vitamins and excretes magnesium from the body.

The following items will help you manage and protect yourself from the stress in your life.

1. **Connect**. Get a strong support system of family and friends around you. When you are having difficult times, feeling a sense of community and belonging helps to dissipate the stress. Not having this, as in my story above, allows everyday stressors to accumulate. Talking things out with others is a woman's pressure-release valve. If you feel isolated or alone, please read the chapter on isolation.

2. **Supplement**. You absolutely *must* make sure you are getting sufficient nutrients to sustain periods of stress. These include increased amounts of B vitamins, magnesium, and easily assimilated Vitamin A. If you are unable to eat a perfect diet (and very few of us are) please make sure to get some high-quality supplements and take them consistently. Food is always the best vehicle to deliver proper nutrition. But from personal experience, I know that times of high-stress usually come with cravings for junk food and oftentimes a lack of availability of healthy food options. Supplement wisely.

3. **Exercise**. Even a ten minute walk can lower cortisol levels and help reset the brain. But if you are able, twenty minute bouts of high-intensity exercise can help to reduce stress more effectively. After all, that's what the stress response is preparing your body to do—fight or flight. On alternate days, try yoga or pilates which helps the body stretch and strengthen while focusing on breathing patterns.

4. **Sleep**. Napping for 20 minutes during the day can do wonders to reset your body. Sleeping in whenever possible also helps during times of duress. In the next chapter on adrenal fatigue, we will discuss this further. But know that your body must have quality sleep at night to reset and recover. **If you are not sleeping well, this is your number one problem to address.** Consider ditching caffeine, sugar, and fried foods from your diet. Add Epsom salt baths to your nighttime ritual. DoTERRA brand Lavender essential oil and/or doTERRA Serenity blend is also helpful when applied to the soles of the feet before bedtime. There are even short yoga routines available online that help stretch the muscles, reset breathing, and quiet the mind for sleep.

5. **Breathe**. Inhale deeply for 5 seconds, hold for 5 seconds, release for 5 seconds. Repeat 5 times. It turns out deep breathing is one of the most powerful and underutilized stress management tools we have. It is easy, and like fasting, requires nothing. Try it out and you will become a believer.

Realize that many of the things we think we need to do every day are not required of us. Sure you have things you must do each day, but staying in a job that robs you of your health, or living in constant fear of paying your mortgage, is optional. If you follow the advice of wise people and accumulate three to six months of living expenses in your savings account, you will have removed large amounts of potential stress from your life. Furthermore, consistently living above your means causes self-inflicted anxiety that you have complete power to eliminate.

Women are amazing in how they care so much for others. Conversely, it is mystifying why most women judge themselves and their own appearance so harshly—usually far more severely than they would ever judge another. The stress that women put upon themselves to live up to unattainable levels of physical perfection is surely a result of the Adversary's plan. He knows that if he can keep you obsessed with your appearance that you will be distracted from doing great things.

Physical beauty comes from within. A happy, healthy woman is far more beautiful than any product of injections and surgery. And know that your self-worth has nothing to do with how you look, but rather with how you think of yourself. We can certainly change our thoughts, even if our physical body is not as accommodating. People are drawn to others because of how they feel around them, not solely because of appearance.

Stress is a monster that must be pro-actively managed or it will take you down. Don't think it will go away on its own. Take the initiative to protect yourself by taking high-quality vitamins and adding nutrient dense foods to safeguard your body. Practice deep breathing every day. Take long walks in nature. Surround yourself with people you love and who add joy to your life.

But if relentless stress has already pushed your body past its limit, adrenal fatigue may be the end result. In the next chapter you will learn how to diagnose, understand, and recover from this often misunderstood disorder.

Chapter 17

ADRENAL FATIGUE:

A Mysterious Malady

Most people have never heard of the adrenals, nor have any idea what they do, even though they are possibly the most over-used organs in our bodies today. The adrenals are walnut-sized glands that sit on top of the kidneys. Their purpose is to make essential hormones that assist our bodies in daily living, reproduction, and coping with stress. However, the highest priority of the adrenals is to ensure survival and help the body return to its natural, balanced state after life-threatening situations.

As part of the endocrine system, these glands work with the thyroid and ovaries in women (and testes in men) to regulate most of the hormonal functions in our bodies. You could think of these three organs as a triangle that rely on each other to communicate needs and regulate the body's energy, endurance, and resiliency. Whenever one of the points of the triangle is weak, the other two points of the triangle attempt to pick up the slack.

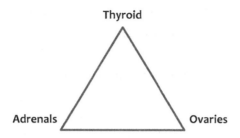

The hormones excreted by the adrenals have many purposes. They dictate how fats and carbohydrates will be used or stored. They instruct the body on when and where to store fat. They dictate blood-pressure by signaling how much sodium will be retained by the body. They determine gastrointestinal function and minimize allergic reactions to protect the body. They create cortisol and epinephrine in response to stressful situations so your body can escape quickly when threatened. They create anti-inflammatory responses when needed to counteract inflammation created by the immune system. They increase or decrease your sex drive. After menopause, women's ovaries go into retirement, and the adrenals manufacture necessary progesterone and estrogen. Additionally, the adrenals secrete hormones that decide your muscle to fat ratio and how long it will take you to recover from a workout.

You have probably heard of athletes taking substances to increase performance. These substances are known as steroids and are naturally created and regulated by the adrenals. It is only when athletes take supplemental steroids that they break the rules of competition. From mass media coverage of the Lance Armstrong case, you are sure to realize steroid abuse is a big deal. It is amazing to think that the hormones created by two tiny glands are so incredibly powerful.

In today's world, stress is an unquestionable daily event. Traffic, work issues, illness, extended family pressures, marriage problems, children's needs, and financial stresses are things we deal with every day. Couple the above with recurring infections, poor diet, lack of sleep, negative thoughts, caffeine, sugar, processed foods, prescriptions, a leaky gut, allergies, and lack of (or excessive) exercise and you have a recipe for adrenal disaster. Constant stressors, like those mentioned above, all take a hit at our adrenals. One by one, they can actually overwhelm our hardest-working glands to the point of exhaustion and dysfunction.

Another issue for women today is the fact that more mothers work and more women are open to the dream of having it all. From personal experience, I've realized that raising children is a full-time job. If you work for yourself or someone else in addition to your family, you are working the equivalent of two to three full time jobs. Having it all is a great idea in theory, but it always comes with a price. Unfortunately more and more women these days are paying that price with their adrenals.

For the average American woman, coffee for breakfast, a high-carb lunch, and a late afternoon pick-me-up coffee with a sugary snack is common. The non-stop list of must-dos everyday often include the following: workout (if you can force yourself to get up early enough), get ready for the day, get kids dressed, fed and off to school or daycare, drop off dry cleaning, make doctor appointments, solve multiple problems at work, meet someone for lunch, run endless errands, pick up kids and take to endless after school activities, help with homework, make dinner, pay bills, do loads of laundry (if you can muster the strength at this point), and then take care of pets and spouse and often other ailing family members. Then, if a woman is lucky, she might get some sleep. The next day it starts all over again, and again, and again.

In my church, the average Latter-day Saint (LDS) woman attempts to prioritize a few more things on her daily task list. We try to pray individually, with our family, and with our spouses. We aim to read our scriptures every day and ponder their contents. We feel the need to assist others in need and help out whenever possible. We hope to hear the influence of the Spirit as we do all these things so that we can be sure to do God's will. We try to do our callings (volunteer church jobs) to the best of our abilities. And we, along with women of all faiths, expect ourselves to do all these things and all the tasks in the above paragraph with grace, 15% body fat, and perfect make-up and hair. Are you starting to notice the plan of the Adversary?

LDS women may not drink coffee, but I have a slew of friends who survive on diet soda or some other form of caffeine to get through the day. Women of all faiths push themselves with over-zealous expectations and often lack time to prepare nutritious meals for themselves and their families. We then resort to take-out food or processed pre-packaged pseudo-food that is devoid of nutrients and good fats. At night we are exhausted but also stressed over all the things that didn't get done. Sleep eludes us.

Then worries and guilt set in over all the things you think you are not doing well. You stress over your weight and lack of exercise regime. You stress over your children and worry about all the problems they have (that you probably blame yourself for). You worry over family, money, health issues, and thing things you haven't achieved or received yet in your life. The list of things to stress over seems endless and sleep does not come. You wake up (or are already awake) when your alarm goes off and start the day exhausted.

Similar to when a newborn has its days and nights mixed up, if you are wired at night and exhausted in the morning, it is a sign of overworked adrenals. The downward spiral of adrenal fatigue can start slowly with a decline in energy and moods. But other times adrenal fatigue symptoms occur abruptly after an intense infection or multiple bouts with an illness. Here are some of the symptoms of adrenal fatigue:

- Difficulty getting up in the morning
- Easily overwhelmed
- Lowered tolerance to annoyances
- Craving for salty foods
- Waking up tired
- Increased PMS
- Low blood pressure
- Less joy with life
- Mild depression
- Sensitivity to cold
- Decreased ability to handle stress
- Brain fog
- Constant need for snacks or caffeine
- Memory loss
- Sensitivity to light
- Needing more effort to achieve same tasks
- Lingering colds that drain all your energy
- Recurring respiratory infections

If you have several of the above symptoms and have been struggling to regain your health, you may have just discovered why recovery has eluded you. Without supporting the adrenals and/or discovering the root cause of the drain on your adrenals, recovery is impossible. So many functions of the female body depend on the adrenals that women are especially vulnerable to a myriad of health issues when the adrenals are not functioning properly.

The Plan of the Adversary

Unfortunately, even though we may be unaware of what our adrenals are and what they do, the Adversary is not. He knows exactly how to sap women of their energy and vitality through constant stress. He also knows that by changing how our food is grown, raised, harvested, and delivered to the public, he can affect the entire population for the worse. Now that you know more about our food supply and how stress affects your body, it is time to learn how to heal your adrenals and recover your energy, vitality, and strength.

The Adrenal Recovery Plan

There are two required steps to restore adrenal health. First, you must discover and remove offending habits and substances that are taxing your adrenal function. Second you must add back in the things your body needs to recover. Basically you must stop the constant drain on the adrenals, and then replenish what has been drained. Note that doing only one step without the other will not allow your adrenals to fully heal.

Step 1: Discover and Remove

Only you can know exactly how certain things make you feel. You are going to have to become more aware of your body and what it is telling you on a daily basis. Once you are able to read the signals your body is sending, you will be able to remove offending substances and situations and finally heal.

Here are some of the things that may be draining your adrenals, your energy, and your health:

Food sensitivities—These often occur after leaky gut syndrome has set in. Discovering the foods that cause your body to react is key to halting stress on the adrenals. Ask a forward-thinking health provider for a food allergy test. Many food sensitivities can be removed by simply avoiding that food for 90 days. Others, such as gluten, may be a lifelong problem. Try re-introducing problem foods one by one after a period of elimination. Monitor any reactions to the food—such as brain fog, clearing of the throat, acid reflux, headaches, joint pain, and intestinal bloating among others—to determine whether you can handle a certain food again.

Not chewing enough while eating—Certain enzymes in your mouth start the digestion process of carbohydrates. If food is not chewed properly, the stomach has to take over the job of carb digestion and is very inefficient. If foods finally reach the small intestine without proper preparation, unwanted bacteria and fungi will feast on the undigested carbohydrates and wreak havoc on the intestines and eventually the rest of the body.

Sugar—Causes a spike in insulin from the pancreas that must be counterbalanced by cortisol created by the adrenals. Cortisol is a stress hormone and too much of it causes weight gain and fatigue. Even worse, eventually the overworked adrenals have trouble keeping up with cortisol production and insulin resistance is the result. If you have adrenal fatigue, sugar and all simple carbohydrates that turn into sugar are not your friends! Ironically you may crave sugar and carbs when your adrenals are overworked. It is a sign of a body out of balance and out of control. You will have to be stronger than the cravings and decide to consciously avoid them for a time to reset your adrenals.

Junk food—Causes a huge drain on your enzyme production factories, your pancreas, and therefore, your adrenals. Avoid like the plague.

Caffeine—Sends emergency signals to your already

overworked adrenals and further drains their scarce resources and capacity.

Pesticides and preservatives—Not only do these toxins get stored away and wreak havoc within our bodies, but because the adrenals control the body's response to allergens, you may become hyper-sensitive to chemicals and additives as a result of out-of-balance adrenals. Eating organic produce and whole foods allows fewer chemicals to potentially set off the allergen alarm, and thus allows the adrenals to rest.

Viruses—Hidden invaders in the form of viruses can keep our immune system on constant alert with little progress to show for it. Viruses literally hide within our cells and fool our immune system by camouflaging themselves. They replicate using our own cell DNA and can be nasty and evasive energy drains on our adrenals.

Parasites—More common than any person would like to admit, parasites are an increasing problem. Because of the sugar, processed food, and lack of nutrients in our diets, our intestinal tracts have become increasingly inviting to invaders. Our normal defense against parasites used to be high levels of stomach acid that kills eggs on contact. Parasites cannot hatch or thrive if their eggs are immobilized before they ever reach our small intestines. But lowered levels of stomach acid from a lack of alkaline vegetables (confusingly, there is an inverse relationship there), leaves you exposed and vulnerable. If the eggs get past this first line of defense, growing parasites then give off toxic wastes that inflame the gut lining and keep your immune system on constant high alert. You may need to consider a parasite cleanse to reclaim your former energy.

Not enough sleep—Your body is in a stress-free state while sleeping. Your body also heals and recovers from past stressors when sleep takes over. Conversely, the more hours you are awake, the harder the adrenals have to work to support your energy levels and the less time they get to recover.

Smoking—Allows dozens of chemicals and toxins to enter your bloodstream. Absolutely avoid at all costs. This includes secondhand smoke.

Prescription and over-the-counter drugs—Contain unfamiliar substances to the body that can set off the adrenal alarm. Avoid whenever possible.

Poor quality water and air—Filtered water is a must. As more and more toxins reach our water supply (including prescription medications, mercury, and lead) community water processing plants are not able to adequately filter out previously unplanned-for particulates. Any and all toxins in our water tax the adrenals. Also, make sure to air out your home and office regularly. Many people do not realize how toxic stagnant, recycled air can be. Houseplants are amazingly efficient at cleaning the air and adding joy to your home. One plant per large room can make a huge difference in air quality. Also consider getting a HEPA air filter for your home and office.

Lack of vitamins and nutrients—Your adrenals absolutely MUST have ample amounts of vitamins and trace minerals to function properly. After adrenal fatigue sets in, you need even higher amounts of these necessary substances to recover.

Constant negative thinking—Causes stress to the body and therefore, sends messages to the adrenals to work harder.

Family or friends who constantly drain your energy—Put a self-imposed barrier between you and these people if at all possible. Unhappy people who drain your energy are taking withdrawals against an already over-drawn account. By removing these energy drains, you allow your health to come first and signal your body to heal.

Toxins in your home or working environment—New

carpet, paint, furniture, draperies, and blinds all contain toxins. Houseplants are the best way to remove many of the off-gassed toxins in our homes and offices. Again, a HEPA air-filter is also helpful.

Not taking time to rest when your body is tired—20 minute naps will do wonders for your adrenals.

Constantly pushing yourself to do and accomplish more—Doing more and more while you have adrenal fatigue is like a hamster trying to run from a cat while on an exercise wheel. You cannot and will not outrun this problem. If you try, the problem will only get worse. (Trust me on this one—I did everything wrong and paid a high price.) Adrenal fatigue is God's way of saying: "Slow down and listen to me. You cannot run faster than you have strength. I am the source of everything you need, and all you have to do is ask." The scripture verse Ether 12:27 in the Book of Mormon truly applies here: "…and I give unto men weakness that they may be humble: and my grace is sufficient for all men that humble themselves before me; for if they humble themselves before me, and have faith in me, then I will make weak things strong unto them."

Living in a state of worry and/or guilt—Worry and guilt are huge energy drains. Often we find that by expressing our worries and issues with another person, that they are not as overwhelming. Talk to someone and put things into proper perspective.

Abuse—No one deserves to be abused—ever. Pray for the courage to seek a change. Pray for the right people to come into your life who will help you remove and overcome abuse.

Step 2: Replenish and Heal

Once you have removed your adrenal "offenders," your next step is to give your body what it needs to heal. Whereas everyone has different sources of stress on the adrenals, the pathway to recovery is the same. Our adrenals need time and tender loving care to recover their former capabilities. Be patient and give yourself time to heal.

The adrenals need the following to recover:

Prayer for help and support—This is always your first step. Make sure to ask for others to pray for you. Be aware that adrenal fatigue may be a call to make changes in your life. Listen to what God, the Universe, the Spirit—whatever can speak to you during this time—has to say. Be willing to give away goals and dreams that aren't leading you to where God wants you to be. Listen, listen, listen. If you encounter any confusion, get advice from people who are closer to the Spirit than you may be capable of being at this time. Get several opinions from trusted sources and weigh their words in your mind before making any major life decisions.

Reframing life stressors—God wants you to know that the only thing you have to do each day is drink water, eat, sleep, breathe, and (hopefully) pray. Everything else is optional. You might ask yourself, "Will this matter in 5, 10, or 20 years?" Or you might ask, "What good am I accomplishing by spending energy stressing over this issue?" My guess is that you might realize you are wasting energy on things you can't control or that ultimately are not important. Let these stressors go and give them to God. He will always prioritize them where they belong.

Good fats—Our adrenals need good fats and healthy amounts of fat-soluble vitamins like A D, E and K to produce hormones, nerve, and cell walls properly. Our Western diets are sadly deficient in good fats and fat-soluble vitamins. Dr. Weston Price found that extremely healthy "primitive" cultures had over 10 times the amount of fat soluble vitamins than the average American diet of the 1930's. The amount of fat-soluble vitamins in today's American diet is most likely worse. Add avocados, organic or preferably raw butter, first-pressed extra-virgin olive oil, and coconut oil to your diet.

Avoidance of fried foods—Fried foods stress the adrenals by causing a need for extra antioxidants to counteract the free-radicals produced from their digestion. Oils used for frying go rancid quickly and are used for days on end in restaurants. The Double Whammy applies here: the more fried foods you eat, the more stress your adrenals incur, plus you forgo the opportunity to eat healthy fats and restore the adrenals. Fried foods are a lose-lose proposition.

Extra Vitamin C—Vitamin C is crucial to all hormones produced by the adrenals. You must get additional Vitamin C to recover from adrenal fatigue as well as to support daily adrenal requirements. The Recommended Daily Allowance of Vitamin C by the US Government is 75-90 mg. Other researchers recommend between 400 and 3000 mg daily to resolve illness and maintain good health. Work with your health care provider to determine the amount of Vitamin C necessary for your recovery. If you are unable to access good health care, try adding 500 mg increments daily to the point your stools become slightly loose. Then remove 500 mg from your dosage. Take this dose daily for at least 3 months. The human body cannot make its own Vitamin C (interestingly, animals can), and we must get this vital nutrient from outside sources. As a result, our bodies adapt to increased amounts received on a daily basis and begin to expect that dosage. Our bodies do not respond as positively to an abrupt decrease in dosage. Do not stop a high dose of Vitamin C abruptly. Taper your dosages down a little each day so your body can adjust and avoid the symptoms of scurvy (severe Vitamin C deficiency). Also note that Vitamin C is water soluble and is removed from the body quickly. <u>Make sure to take doses several times per day in order to heal.</u>

Orange juice has too much natural sugar to be a helpful source of Vitamin C. Furthermore, as orange juice sits on a shelf over the winter, the Vitamin C loses its potency. The insulin spike and consequent adrenal demand from drinking orange juice is not worth the small Vitamin C benefit. Eat citrus fruits in their natural form or juice them yourself for maximum nutritional impact.

Extra sleep—The more you rest, the quicker your adrenals will recover. However, sleep may be difficult as a burst of energy at bedtime is common, as well as insomnia. Try 2-5 mgs of melatonin at night to aid a deep, restful sleep. A high protein snack with good fats before bed can help balance out blood sugar and keep you from waking in the middle of the night. Exercise in the morning also helps you sleep deeper at night. You may need hormone assistance to regulate your sleep patterns. (Personally, I had to get on bio-identical progesterone before I could sleep properly.) Also try to go to bed before 10:30 pm and sleep in until 9 am whenever possible. Sleeping from 6-9 am is especially restorative. Trade kids with a trusted friend or family member and sleep in!

A good multivitamin twice a day—This is an absolute necessity to support all the other functions for which the adrenals are trying to compensate.

Gentle exercise—Intense exercise is not a good idea when your adrenals are sapped. It utilizes vitamin and mineral stores that are already depleted. During intense exercise, these glands are required to make even more hormones to sustain super-high energy needs and recovery. Yoga, pilates, walking, swimming, and light jogging are all good choices to gently rebuild the adrenals. Yoga is *especially* beneficial as it also allows the brain to reboot. Doing yoga allows the body to downgrade stress and worry to more manageable levels. Yoga also loosens the muscles and ligaments and literally slows the process of aging by releasing toxins and past injuries. Yoga is a great friend to adrenal recovery and overall health.

Laughter—Laughing literally heals the body. Stress cannot exist simultaneously with laughter. Watch funny, uplifting shows or listen to clean comedians in your car or on your iPod. Make an effort to laugh heartily several times a day.

Adrenal support supplements—Talk with your doctor about support supplements. There are many good formulas to support the adrenals available today. As more and more people learn about adrenal fatigue, the market for these products allows higher quality and better combinations to reach consumers. Some that I have tried with good results are Adrenoplex by Priority One, or Adrenal Medulla by Allergy Research Group paired with Adaptocrine by Apex Energetics. Make sure to get the advice of a trusted health professional on which dosages to use for your particular situation.

Free time to get lost in something you love—Can you remember when you were a child and could get lost in a beloved activity for hours? You didn't think about anything you "had" to do, you just played. Well, you just got a free pass to recreate that type of situation. You must carve out time to do something you love. Life is not enjoyable when all we do is work, stress, and toil. God never meant for you to live a life devoid of joy. Go find what makes you happy and spend some time doing it! Find a babysitter, set an appointment with yourself on your calendar, and get your spouse on board that you need this to heal. Your adrenals will respond to your joy and heal all the faster.

Final Considerations

Recovering from adrenal fatigue takes time. It is difficult for women to slow down and take care of themselves because we are programmed to take care of the needs of others. The more you allow yourself to rest, the faster you will heal. Enlist the help of others and allow them to receive the blessings of serving you. In the end, how fast you recover is all up to you.

Something else to note: many people I have encountered with adrenal fatigue are Type-A, overachiever, highly-driven, goal-oriented types. While being passionate and driven are both wonderful characteristics, they are also physically draining characteristics. Make sure you support your drive with healthy eating, only the best fats, little to no sugar, and supplements, or you may find yourself sitting on the sidelines. If you do find yourself on a forced "time-out," make sure you try to listen to the Spirit to help you prioritize your daily activities. Every woman I know has way too many things to accomplish on her daily task list—and I realize these tasks do not disappear when you are ill. Only Heavenly Father knows which tasks are *truly* important in our eternal progression, and He is happy to help guide us whenever we ask.

Chapter 18
TAKING OFFENSE AND GETTING OVER IT

From watching women in the workplace, in their homes, at church, and at school, I have noticed patterns of behavior that are undeniable. Women want to belong and feel accepted. They also want to love, serve, create, provide, and protect—but above all, we want to belong. The possibility of being left out or specifically excluded affects our actions and choices. Every woman has been excluded at some point in her life. Usually in junior high or even earlier, we experienced being excluded by other girls or worse, close friends turned against us. It's not a feeling you forget quickly. Some women are more able to forgive and move on, while others are changed forever by the experience. The deciding factor between these two events comes down to several things including insecurities, hormones, and thought patterns.

Every human being is insecure about something: appearance, weight, job status, marriage status, number of kids, cooking ability, number of wrinkles, grey hair, what you haven't accomplished, what you don't own, spirituality level, lovability, number of friends, lack of education, speaking ability, creativity levels, and more. Women are just programmed to be more aware of their shortcomings than men. Women of faith are even more mindful of what we lack because we are trying to follow Christ and are very aware we fall woefully short. Because we live in an imperfect world, we are subject to Satan's constant barrages of pointing out our inadequacies according to the world's standards. Then we turn around and realize we are a long way off from reaching the Lord's requirements, too. No matter which way we turn, it can become painfully obvious that we are a long way from anywhere.

Satan focuses his efforts on women to keep guilt and our insufficiencies at the forefront of our minds. He wants to keep us just distracted enough so that we are unable to achieve great things. He realizes that he can't keep us from doing good things, or even perhaps "better" things—but he will do all he can to keep you from doing the best things. He accomplishes this through a constant attack on our self-esteem. Usually through our own negative thoughts, we beat ourselves up over every "should have" and "could have" along with a complete disdain of our appearance. Add in a poor diet (mostly unknowingly), lack of exercise, poor sleep, and too much stress and eventually the negative thoughts erode our health and self-esteem like a parasite.

Being over-stressed, hormonally bankrupt and insecure makes any woman an easy target for being offended. All it takes is another person to push one of our insecurity "buttons" for the fireworks to fly. Anytime there is a conflict of considerable measure among women, you can guarantee one if not both parties have hit the other's insecurity buttons. Imagine the scenario like this: You enter an elevator that has a least twenty floor buttons followed by an unknown small child; you are in a hurry to get to the 20th floor; the child presses the entire wall of buttons and says "Pretty!" while you try not to explode. Now imagine the small child has just turned into your personal button-pusher. Can you relate to having one of those in your life?

Once a woman's buttons are pushed, a few things can potentially happen. One—she can come out swinging; two—she can wrangle her anger into a state of passive-aggressive behavior and secret loathing of the other person; three—she can go home and cry and wonder why that person was so mean to her; four—she can shut the other person out of her life forever; or five—she can give the other person the benefit of the doubt and try not to let it bother her.

The true final result of a disagreement depends on how capable a woman is of "letting things go." Some are better at it than others. Those who perceive arguments as a normal part of life are better equipped to resolve things quickly. Other women cannot bounce back without considerable time and prayer. Some women can't seem to recover at all. Bear in mind, just because you get over things quickly does not mean others have that same gift.

If we can be vulnerable enough to realize our own insecurities, we could change the world. We would be aware of situations that push our buttons and seek help to overcome these feelings. Being courageous enough to be vulnerable is an act of faith. Acting to improve on what you learn about yourself is the next step. Dr. Brené Brown wrote an entire book on vulnerability and why we avoid it. In her book, *Daring Greatly,* she explores the difference between people who feel a deep sense of love and belonging and those who struggle for it and came to this conclusion: "That one [difference] was the belief in their worthiness [to be loved and belong]." [47]

As believers in a higher power and our divine origin, we women of faith need to really *believe* the phrase: We are daughters of our Heavenly Father, who loves us, and we love Him. If this statement truly resonated with each of us and we understood our divine nature to our very core, we would never take offense. We would be completely happy with our authentic self. There would be no need for competition or insecurity because none of the Adversary's lies would ring true to us.

All the temptations to which we are exposed are chocolate-covered lies: putting others down will make us feel better, contention "clears the air," or by being perfect you will be beyond reproach. Dr. Brown calls perfection the 20-ton shield and explains it is what people do to avoid scrutiny by their peers. These people's greatest fear is being found unworthy or unacceptable by others. Unfortunately, perfection also keeps the person in glittery box, unable to present their true self and talents to the world.

Hormones are another factor in why women take offense. It does not matter how positively you try to think or live your life, if your hormones are out of whack—so is your ability to gracefully accept the blows life dishes out. Balance your hormones, and you will find a new world waiting for you. From personal experience of years of hormonal upheaval, offenses came much more readily than when compared to my hormone-balanced youth.

A friend of mine told me how she and her husband had knock-down-drag-out fights for years. She lived in fear that their marriage was crumbling and her family would be ripped apart. Finally one day, her husband asked her when her monthly cycle started. He began to track her cycles on his own. He figured out every month right before her period started they would get in a huge fight. He had even mapped it on a calendar for himself. Once she realized this (after he wisely braved the conversation with her on a less hormone-ridden day), she was so relieved their marriage wasn't in danger that she laughed herself silly. She realized that during these times she would get offended by something her husband would say or assume he meant and start a fight. It happened like clockwork. She later sought out help, and her husband supported her whole-heartedly.

Hormones are vicious and necessary evils in this world. If we all lived in a toxin-free, nutrient-dense, stress-free world, our hormones would work perfectly. Unfortunately, we do not live in this kind of perfect world. Countless women become different people throughout their hormonal ups and downs. Some of us realize it and try to hold in the carnage, while others either cannot or aren't aware enough to realize their hormones are ruling their lives.

Your hormones affect how deeply something hurts you—whether perceived or real. They also determine recovery time and how you will store the memory—as an unpleasant event or something to be avoided in the future at all costs. When something happens that causes you great pain, your adrenals produce epinephrine which signals the body is in great danger. This same hormone allows the memory of that event to sear itself into the cells of your brain. If your body is out of balance and cannot signal to the brain that things are resolved in a sufficient amount of time, the event may remain registered as a much larger danger than it actually was. In this manner, we collectively store thousands of experiences and how they made us feel. We store our thoughts and feelings and match them with a response. These experiences determine how we will react in the future.

We may not even understand why certain situations cause strong emotions within us. For example, for years whenever my father would call to catch up, he would always ask me how my little sister was doing. For some reason, this angered me every time. I would think, "I don't know—why don't you ask her? Why are you always asking me about her like I am her mother? Did you call to talk to me or find out what's going on in her life?" I realized this situation angered me, but I didn't know exactly why. It made no sense. I was a married adult with children and had a great relationship with my sister. I loved her and wanted only the best for her. Why this situation angered me remained a mystery to me for decades. Through a blessed personal connection, I found a process called resonance repatterning that helped me understand why I reacted with anger in that situation. I will reveal the reason and the process in the next chapter.

Have you ever heard the expression: "People may not remember what you say, but they will never forget the way you made them feel?" That is because the *emotion* created from either the positive or negative experience you have with someone is stored differently in the brain. That memory is accessed differently, and remains sharp and clear. Other memories, like simple conversations for example, are not stored for quick retrieval because they did not invoke a strong emotional response.

Our thought patterns also play a large part in how easily offended we are. Unmet expectations—perhaps set unrealistically high on someone else—can trigger hurt feelings. After all is said and done, I have realized one tenet of truth that holds its own for the vast majority of people. This tenet helps me to give people the benefit of the doubt, avoid offense, and save myself a lot of doubt and suffering. I hope it will help you as well. The tenet is this:

The vast majority of people do not intend to hurt you.

They may be selfish, clueless, or narcissistic but they do not set out to hurt you on purpose. Ask yourself this question: Did that person really intend to hurt me by saying or doing that? If the answer is an honest no, it makes it easier not to take things personally.

If you give others the benefit of the doubt that they had a hard day, a bad childhood, or are achingly insecure, you are enabled to forgive them or perhaps avoid offense in the first place. If something happens that enrages you, give it some time before you do or say anything. Your hormones may be driving some strong emotions that will subside with time. Once you can see things logically, without being overwhelmed with emotion—which happens to all women whether we admit it or not—the entire situation can change like patterns in a kaleidoscope.

On the other hand, if someone has a history or pattern of inflicting pain on you, you have your free agency to remove them from your life. Jesus said we had to love everyone, he didn't say we had to endure unending abuse. You can love and forgive someone from afar. Just make sure you get the opinion of several people you trust before removing a spouse or close family member from your life. Be very honest with yourself and make sure you take responsibility for your part of the problem. If you don't correct your own behavior, you may find yourself in a similar situation in the future. Like attracts like. This is where resonance repatterning can be greatly beneficial. We will discuss it at length in the next chapter.

Chapter 19
RESONANCE REPATTERNING:
Healing the Hidden Wounds

Through years of searching for answers to my health problems, I was lead from one health provider to another for specific reasons of which I was not aware at the time. Each one of the doctors, naturopaths, chiropractors, and applied kinesiologists I met added a piece to the puzzle.

Even my husband was part of the path. For years he had been battling sinus headaches which had morphed into aches and pains throughout his upper body. He was in pain every day with no relief. Through his own research he began to wonder if he had contracted Lyme disease. He found a naturopathic doctor in Austin, Texas, who once suffered from Lyme disease herself. Dave went to visit her, and I soon followed. She was a great help to my husband and then to me. At the very least, we were both able to rule out Lyme disease through a series of specialized lab tests. The best part was that she was humble and open to the fact the she may not be able to heal us entirely.

In a personal consultation for me alone, this doctor went

through a long list of other processes and practitioners that might be worth looking into. As I listened intently to her referral suggestions, one option in particular resonated with me. This option was a local practitioner who was trained in a process called Resonance Repatterning. She explained that repatterning helped to re-set emotional traumas in the body which would allow the body to heal physically.

It sounded completely whacked out and hokey. But I couldn't deny that I had past experiences that had not been resolved. I carried the memories of certain events as if they happened yesterday, and the difficulty of my pregnancies and the resulting postpartum depression had left deep pains etched in my soul. I still felt that God had abandoned me at the most painful and difficult time of my life. It felt like I had open wounds that my body was exhaustedly trying to keep from infection—the wounds just happened to be emotional.

At this point in my health journey, I began to reexamine my earlier stance of thinking physical issues were keeping me from healing emotionally. I began to wonder if I had reached a new layer which needed attention. And I questioned whether certain emotions were now keeping me from healing physically, and how the two states interacted.

At this time I had extreme brain fog and lack of patience with my children. I felt depleted and downtrodden every day. I was constantly exhausted and my monthly cycles caused mood rollercoasters of epic proportions. I knew instinctively that the mother sets the tone of a household. Her love, moods, energy levels and spirituality affect every person in the home to an immeasurable degree. Having had the blessing of a kind and loving mother, I knew I was nowhere near being the balanced and consistent mom my children deserved. I could tell my children were starting to react to my impatience, anger, and constant stressed-out state with fear and wariness of me. I had held back my emotions for so long and tried to protect them in their innocent years but my veneer and my health was starting to wear thinner and thinner. I didn't want them to grow up being scared of their sick mother who was unpredictable and incapable of helping them with their own problems. I knew something had to change, and for their sakes, I was willing to try anything—hokey or not.

I started my research at www.repatternit.com. On the website, patients describe their initial problems and how repatterning helped them overcome their issue. One woman on the website described how her constant anger and anxiety was affecting her child and how being repatterned changed the entire dynamic of their home for the better. It resonated so strongly with me I finally got the courage to call Mary Schneider and make an appointment.

The first time I went to see Mary I was not sure what to expect. We started with a whole lot of talking and as we chatted Mary flicked her forefinger and thumb against one another as she looked over one of her books. When I asked her about it she explained she was muscle testing for which area we needed to work on that day.

I was first exposed to muscle testing when I went to an applied kinesiologist and chiropractor years before. It is a process where you ask a yes or no question while testing the resistance of a particular muscle. If the answer is yes the muscle will hold strong, if the answer is no the muscle will not be able to hold the resistance. The premise is that your spirit knows all things if we would only ask. It seemed really hokey to me at first, like the chiropractor was just making things up and pressing harder on my arm to get a yes answer. It was a lot like having faith in Christ—it can seem like a bunch of nonsense that other people believe to make themselves feel better. But after many experiences with muscle testing

I began to realize that it really worked—in spite of my disbelief. That was my first foray away from traditional western medicine. I was not easily swayed from all that I had learned from my childhood about doctors and conventional medicine. But since they had not helped me get well in spite of me putting all my faith in them, I had no choice but to seek other options.

Muscle testing only works if the person facilitating the testing is healthy, balanced, and able to tap into their own spirit. The person being tested also needs to be somewhat physically healthy with respect to having strength in the muscles used for the test. During my health struggles the doctor often had a tough time finding a muscle that was consistently strong enough to test with. I now realize this was because I was not only physically unwell but completely out of touch with the Spirit. I had consciously disconnected because I felt I had been abandoned in my time of greatest need. I realized I could never have trusted any muscle testing I conducted on myself or anyone else at that time because I didn't trust my own instincts. I was very much out of balance.

After a minute of testing, Mary would explain what area was showing as needing repatterning. This test would uncover the area of the body or energetic system that related to the issue I was having. The process uses a myriad of different modalities including color, light, movement, music, the ayurvedic chakra system, the Chinese 5-element acupuncture system, cranial sacral work and many other healing modalities. Certified Resonance Repatterning practitioners are trained in all these healing modalities and are able to apply them when needed.

For those of you who are rolling your eyes right now, I completely understand. If I had not personally been driven to a place of little hope, I would have never believed any of this for a second. I was a left-brained, math and economics type with zero belief in things you cannot prove (except for God, who I believed in implicitly, even when I thought He had abandoned me). Furthermore, growing up in the LDS faith I was taught to be suspicious of those things that would cause contention, confusion, and drive away the Spirit. There was a constant warning mechanism in my brain for all things new-age and hippie-esque.

I also realized that going to any kind of emotional counselor required one to be completely vulnerable and open to influence in order for healing to occur. If I went to a counselor who had unresolved personal issues, was easily offended, or vehemently disagreed with my personal beliefs—whether openly or covertly, I could potentially be swayed away from my true center because of the influence they held over me at such a vulnerable time. All of these issues had to be resolved before I would fully open myself to the experience.

Fortunately for me, Mary was the perfect mix of healer, guide, and respecter of my beliefs. After testing and watching her responses I could perceive that she had no hidden agenda against religion or others' beliefs. I could tell she did not get offended by anything I believed or said which showed how healthy and balanced she was. She was kind without being overly empathetic, helpful without being a crutch, and never pushed for additional sessions (which is a huge red flag for me). The session itself not only re-sets the frequency of a wrongly held belief (such as "I am unworthy of love," or "If I become successful, people I love will tear me down," or "There is not enough for me to share") but was a two hour therapy session where I could speak freely and be heard. So many people today just need to be heard!

I had gone to LDS counselors several times in previous years. One was especially amazing at explaining shame, guilt, and notions of inadequacy. She was able to frame it perfectly within the gospel and opened my eyes to how many of us live with unbearable guilt and shame. But even working with her for many months did not change the way I felt—it only made me aware of *why* I felt that way. Working with Mary actually changed the way I felt.

I share the following experience with you in the hopes that it will shed light and understanding on the process of Resonance Repatterning and open your mind to other methods of healing. If we are to truly heal, we have to find the source of the trouble and fix it. Here is how just one repatterning awakened my understanding of the anger issues I had towards my father and sister (that were mentioned in the previous chapter); issues I had carried all my life and never understood—and how the issue was resolved.

A Big Awakening

One overcast weekday I found myself lying on my back at my repatterning appointment, wondering what we would work on that day. The pleasantries of greeting were over, and Mary muscle tested for what area needed re-setting. She announced, "I'm coming up with the heart meridian repatterning which deals with healing a broken heart and issues of control. I'm also showing that it has something to do with you and your mother when you were 3 years old." She asked if I knew of anything that happened between us during that time. I, of course, don't remember being three years old, let alone anything that happened at that age but then it came to me. "My sister was born that year," I said.

Mary began to ask me a series of questions from her guidebook on the heart meridian and muscle tested me to see if the yes or no questions resonated with me. Examples of these statements are: Who is it difficult for you to open your heart to? What quality in that person makes it difficult for you to open your heart? What quality in you makes it difficult for you to open your heart to that person?

After answering some specific questions for Mary, I began to realize a pattern of behavior I had displayed my entire life. I had always been overly annoyed by my little sister: when she cried as an infant, when she wanted to play with me as a toddler, when she wanted to borrow my clothes in junior high, when she wanted to be friends with my friends in high school. I remember admitting to myself that I was afraid that she would grow up to be more beautiful and popular than me and that when that happened, I would fade into nothingness. My mother would tell me I was being very selfish to not share my things with her, and so I began to view myself as selfish and stubborn but didn't care. I wasn't going to share anything of mine with her if I could help it—not ever.

As adults, my sister and I became very good friends, and most of my "selfishness" subsided. But as I mentioned previously, when my father would call me and ask me about my sister, I would get incensed and never understood why. While Mary walked me through the series of questions I realized that I must have been somewhat neglected when my infant sister arrived and formulated a belief in my 3-year old mind that my sister took away my mother's and father's love and attention from me. I began to resent her arrival from that time forward.

Never would I have realized this fact through my own

memory—it was deeply protected in the depths of my mind after being created by my 3-year old self. But as I thought about my behavior throughout my life towards my sister, it all started to make perfect sense. My mother had even recently told me that during that time she would get the baby down and then my older brother, but by the time she got to me I had already fallen asleep. She admitted she had felt badly for not being able to give me more attention. Mary proceeded to reset the wrong belief I held and helped to fill that void with positive beliefs of self-worth and self-acceptance. She role-played my mother and apologized to me for that time period where she couldn't give me more attention. We then did some work with color and sound to reset the resonance of my old belief.

I am not going to lie to you, I left that day feeling like an emotional train wreck. I had two distinct physical reactions over the next hours and days. Immediately upon leaving her office, I felt a pain in my right mid-abdomen start to move to the left that felt like a stone of grief being passed. Secondly, the next 24 hours consisted of a pure sadness that only a child can feel. It was simple and uncomplicated and extremely heavy to bear. I cried and felt the pain that I had stored away and refused to face so long ago. I told myself to be brave and just let the feelings come. It was a somber night. The following day, I felt the sadness lift and looked at the clock—it was 11:03 am. Almost exactly 24 hours had passed since I left Mary's office. I was amazed at how the sadness had dissipated—it was simply gone.

For several days I experienced intestinal issues as it felt like the "stone of grief" passed through my system. After about five days, this also dissipated and did not return. I learned later that resentment is held in the gallbladder and anger is held in the liver. It made perfect sense to have the symptoms I had.

The mother of one of my best friends was molested by a church member when she was 8 years old. When she tried to tell someone about her abuser, they did not believe her. She did not see a therapist about the repeated abuse until much later in life. She has endured many health problems and has had 2 liver transplants. Her justifiable anger towards her abuser and not being believed when she came forward has affected her body her entire life. Our emotions can absolutely compromise our internal organs and energy levels. Negative emotions held for years can decimate a person's health. Don't let past abuses fester in your soul. You deserve to feel peace. Seek out a counselor or friend you can confide in, or better yet, get repatterned. You may be holding onto past emotions and not even realize it.

What I learned from this experience is that we can each create and hold onto negative or untrue thoughts throughout our lives. Through abuse or neglect we often begin to think we are unlovable or unworthy of good things. We may not even realize we have created and housed this negative belief. These beliefs can manifest themselves as self-sabotage, negative patterns of behavior, or anger and rage in our adult lives. For me, it was created by a 3 year-old's untrue perception of her surroundings.

Have you ever noticed that when left uninformed of a situation, little children will come to the worst possible conclusion about themselves? Children assume they are to blame for a myriad of parental problems: anger issues, abuse, exhaustion, divorce, neglect. Their innocent little minds are incapable of placing blame on anyone other than themselves. It is one of their sweetest qualities and an indicator of the purity and intensity of their love.

Thinking of little children who are hurt and neglected breaks my heart. My hope is that every mother and father will have a chance to heal his or her own physical, mental, and emotional weaknesses before they are passed on to their children. Kids repeat their parents' behavior when they grow up and start to raise their own children. We can tell our children how to do something correctly, but if we are not patterning that behavior for them it is unlikely our words will take hold within them.

Resonance repatterning allows men and women to let go of their wrongly held beliefs and embrace the good in life. Negative patterns of behavior can be understood and reset quickly. I have been to many sessions and am always amazed at how timely and insightful the day's work is. For the record, only two sessions caused uncomfortable physical results afterwards—and the final results I experienced made the sadness and intestinal discomfort worth every second.

I no longer feel a simmering anger towards my father or sister, and even more importantly I realized I am not a selfish person. My actions were a direct result of an underlying untrue belief I had created that has now been corrected. Mary is an excellent facilitator but takes no credit for herself. She simply "follows the process" to where it leads. I know that process is directed by the Spirit who is always ready to help those who ask for it.

You may wonder why faith and prayer alone could not resolve these issues. The answer is: because you don't know the issue exists. The human mind has the innate ability to protect us from pain and suffering by storing emotions or memories behind locked doors, so to speak. In order to conquer that fear, and forgive others when necessary, you must face it at some point. Your human mind will protect you as long as it can, but at some point the pain starts to break through and wear away at your character and health.

We were allowed to come to earth to learn and to help each other. If you were to be divinely healed without understanding what wound existed in the first place, you would miss out on an important learning experience. For some, to be a guide or facilitator in helping others overcome their afflictions is a divine calling and a blessing. We each have the opportunity to learn from our mistakes and to help guide others through the process. My alcoholic friend who assists others starting their own alcoholism recovery shared that so many people just need someone to hold their hand through the unknown. Fear and uncertainty are overwhelming deterrents to asking for help. Without leaning into the initial fear, we are incapable of being helped and making the needed changes.

Heavenly Father can only help us if we will offer up our fears to Him and let Him remove them. The process truly requires courage. One woman recently shared her frustration with God for not eliminating a certain character flaw even after many fervent and sincere prayers for help. When she could quiet her mind to hear His response, it was, "You have to release your grasp so I can take it from you." Sometimes we need help to realize what we are desperately clutching so we can let it go.

Resonance Repatterning can be done in person or by proxy over the phone. It is also known as Holographic Repatterning. You can search for a local practitioner in your area through the internet or contact Mary through her website at www.repatternit. com. I wish you the very best as you face your own demons. Be brave and pray for courage! It is worth every short-lived discomfort to be able to let go of your fears and truly live.

Chapter 20
COMPROMISED THOUGHTS AND MENTAL MAINTENANCE

I'm worried about my friend, Gretchen. It's as if she has become a different person. She's thinking of leaving her husband and kids. She's started drinking and says she doesn't believe in anything spiritual anymore. We used to serve together in church. What can I do to help her?

Have you ever encountered a situation like this? I'm hearing it happen more and more every day. Good men and women making terrible decisions and leaving huge amounts of pain and despair in their wake. Decisions to turn away from what brings true happiness are becoming all too common. I believe this often occurs because of depression and other physical illnesses. I hope that by shedding light on the lies of the Adversary you can help yourself and others out of the vicious cycle of a compromised physical body believing spiritual lies which leads to even more physical illness.

Spiritual Untruths

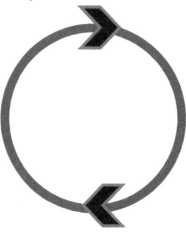

Physical Imbalances

Our minds are very, very powerful. "For as he thinketh in his heart, so is he." (Proverbs 23:7) False beliefs about our self-worth have caused many men and women throughout this mortal existence to suffer great anguish of the soul. Women have left their children thinking they would be better off without them. Men have abandoned their families thinking they just weren't cut out to be fathers. Children make a poor choice, are told they are bad, and then believe it the rest of their lives. And these examples don't even begin to include the vast number of people who are abused, neglected and instilled with feelings of little to no self-worth from a very young age.

Sometimes our poor choices come from a lack of understanding or experience. Other times, they may come from another source altogether. From my own experience, and from searching for answers on the body and how it functions, I have come to realize that many, many people suffer from depression, hormone issues, chemical imbalances, and sickness that affect the decisions they make on a large scale.

Here are some examples of spiritual untruths that if believed, can potentially cause physical imbalances or be more easily believed in the presence of physical illness and imbalance:

Spiritual Untruth

You will never be good enough.
You are unlovable.
You are nothing.
You have no talents.
The world would be better off without you.
You are a failure.
It is all your fault.
Everyone else can do it—why can't you?
You are worthless.
You'll never make a decent living.
You will always be unpopular.
You don't fit in here.
You are not wanted.
You have no self-control because you always overeat.
You are not chosen.
You are unclean.
You are broken.
You are not smart enough.
You can never clean-up the messes you've made.

Messages like these bombard everyone at some point in their lives. They are all falsehoods forged by the Father of All Lies, and can only affect us if we believe them and let them take root in our consciousness. If they do take root, they cause stress and misery that affects us physically and mentally.

On the other side of the cycle, I know that depression,

hormones, imbalanced brain chemistry, food allergies, and chronic pain and inflammation can lead us to believe many spiritual untruths about our abilities and self-worth. Remember, Satan loves to kick us when we are down. A time of illness is the perfect time for him to assault an otherwise un-moveable soul. And if our bodies become sick enough, we can find ourselves on a downward spiral of destruction and despair.

For example, I know a couple who were high school sweethearts, married in the temple and were blessed with several children. Life was good for them—they got along well, he made a good living, she was able to stay home with the kids, and the family was happy and healthy. The husband, whom we'll call Brian, decided he wanted to get into better physical shape. He went on a 900 calorie per day diet and worked out like a fiend. He got very, very fit. But after a few months on his new fitness regime, his family didn't seem to bring him joy anymore. He started to lose interest in his wife and decided he had never loved her. Soon thereafter, he told her he wanted a divorce. She was stunned and shocked. What had happened to her husband? Where had his former self gone?

The truth is he depleted his body of many vital fats, vitamins and minerals during his extreme diet and workout regime that he did not replace properly. This affected the serotonin, dopamine, and GABA levels in his brain. He became mentally and physically run down and spiritual disconnection was the result. It wasn't that his family didn't bring him joy any longer; it was that *nothing* brought him joy anymore. He was chemically imbalanced and unwell. The temptations of the Adversary became harder and harder to fight or even to figure out why was he fighting them in the first place. It seemed as if his very soul—the essence of his former self—was thinning with each passing day, like a bed sheet that is becoming threadbare, and then finally translucent. The reality was that his spirit had not disappeared; it was just temporarily silenced by a broken mind and body. He needed physical help to heal his body so he could reconnect with his spirit.

Our bodies are the vessels that we are given to maneuver our spirits through this life. As mentioned in a previous chapter, our mortal experience is optimized when we use our spirit to drive our body. Heavenly Father wants us to connect with Him and be happy. Unfortunately, the Adversary doesn't want us to know that our spirits can be in control. He wants our easily influenced and imperfect body to drive. He feeds us lies that we must fight against in order to accomplish our divine plan on this earth. He tempts us with things that would bind us in chains of addiction and despair. Additionally, over the last few decades the Adversary has influenced man to affect our food supply and popular eating traditions in attempts to malnourish and confuse the mind. He knows that if he can break down our bodies and minds, our spirits will be trapped in vessels of depression, illness, and immobility.

To win in today's world, we have to swim upstream. You may not be able to swim quickly. You might be broken, exhausted and have little hope—but you have more strength than you realize. All that is required of you is to keep trying. Disbelieve commonly accepted nutrition practices. Disconnect from the constant barrage of advertisements with hidden agendas. Hold onto your faith. As you swim against the tide of popular nutritional fallacies and beliefs, disparaging media messages on physical perfection, and the disdain or apathy of others towards religion and spirituality you will start to see the lies of the Adversary for what they are—distractions from true happiness.

As a Woman Thinketh

I am a big believer in personal responsibility. We will all be held accountable for our choices and one day everyone will be judged for their own actions. But what if some of the things that influenced your poor decisions were beyond your control? By way of example, suppose you learned years afterwards that you didn't do well in school because you had a learning disability, and that all the years of pain you spent thinking you were unintelligent were unfounded. What if Brian's wife learned he left the family because he had mental and physical health issues instead of thinking that it was her fault? Revealed truth about previously misunderstood circumstances can lift age-old heartaches.

What thoughts do you think the Adversary would prefer you to hold onto? My guess is any thought that causes you misery. What if, instead, you simply let those thoughts go? Instead of finding familiarity and comfort in those old pains, you chose to alter your perspective on things. Like the kaleidoscope mentioned in the chapter on taking offense, I have found that when you look at something just slightly differently, the entire picture can change.

So how do we turn around our darkest thoughts and stop our suffering? One of the best methods I have encountered is called "The Work" by Byron Katie. After years of misery, she had a revelation wherein she realized that suffering is optional. The result of her experience is a method of inquiry that is simple and powerful. Basically, you ask yourself if the thought which causes you pain is correct. Can you absolutely, positively know without a doubt that the thought is accurate? If not, you might be better off without it.

For example, having grown up with a weight problem, I often felt ugly next to my friends. Even after losing weight, I still saw myself as unattractive. Was I truly dreadful-looking? I sure thought so. But could I know without a doubt that that was really, truly accurate? No, not really. Furthermore, when I believed that I was unattractive, I felt sad and distant from others. But without that thought, I felt free and no longer obsessed over my appearance. I could then focus all that mental energy in a more positive direction.

Byron Katie further explains that we experience pain when we mentally get into other people's business. She clarifies that there are only three people in the world whose business you can be in: your own, other people's, and God's. When you are thinking or worrying about anybody else's business than your own, you are inviting pain and worry into your mind. No one can live someone else's life for them; that is their business. And no one knows when or how war and weather catastrophes will strike; that is God's business. When you let go of mental worry and strife over things you have no control over, you free your mind to focus on your own life and take action on things you can control.

Katie has several books with multiple examples of how she walks individuals through their most painful beliefs: *Loving What Is*, *Who Would You Be Without Your Story?*, *I Need Your Love - Is That True?*, *A Thousand Names For Joy*, and *Question Your Thinking, Change The World*. She assists people not only in exposing their untrue beliefs, but in turning them around to see the greater truth. By realizing that it is not our experiences that cause us pain, but the thoughts we assign to them, we are free to shed the light of truth on these thoughts and release them. You can learn more about "The Work" at Katie's website, www.thework. com, and by doing an exercise called "Judge your neighbor."

When you understand what causes your painful thoughts, you can experience respite and joy. Even if our negative thoughts are influenced by imbalances and illness, we can realize we have a choice in what we believe. We can be gentle with ourselves if there were times when our decisions were difficult to make. When we *know* better, we can *do* better. By understanding that the thoughts we have about ourselves and others are not necessarily true, we have the opportunity to cast aside suffering and not pass it on to others. We have the power within us to break chains of misery passed down through generations. Get off the downward spiral of believing lies leading to illness leading to succumbing to more deceit. I pray that you will harness this power in your own life. When you do, you will become a source of light and joy to the world.

In the next chapters we will discuss how to heal your body when you have tried everything else, but the sadness still overwhelms you. These are cases where isolation and depression must be addressed.

Chapter 21

ISOLATION:

How to Break the Cycle

You're standing in a crowd and you've never felt so alone. You're at a church activity and feel like you can't relate to anyone there. You see other people on Facebook posting pictures of the runs they did with friends or the group dinners they enjoy but you have nothing to post. You see neighbors all around you getting together but you're not invited. You move to a new place and want to get to know people but are too afraid to "get out there" so you sit at home night after night. You tell yourself you don't want to get netted in to the drama and neediness of others so you protect yourself by pulling into your own protective shell.

You're isolated. You feel it. You know it. But you don't know how to fix it or if you even want to.

If you are longing for more interaction with others to the point where it brings you great sadness, there is an imbalance in your life—a big one. Most people experience this longing to some degree at some point in their lives. No one is immune to loneliness. Humans are meant to be together. We are genetically programmed to need interaction with others. It does not matter whether you are an introvert who derives energy from being alone, or an extrovert who is energized by being around others— we all need human interaction.

Spiritually, you have been surrounded by brothers and sisters for eternities before you came to earth. When you were born into your earthly body, you were descended from generations of families and tribes who banded together to survive. No one was born to be alone. It is not in our spiritual or physical DNA.

Just like the physical imbalances that lead to spiritual imbalances and back around again, there is a circular pattern to the causes and circumstances that breed feelings of isolation:

The Isolation Cycle

Depression

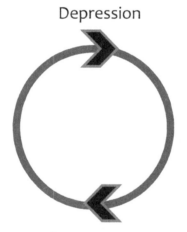

Lack of Human Interaction

When my oldest daughter was almost a year old, my husband got a job offer in Austin, Texas. Even though I was sick and rarely felt in-tune with God, I felt strongly that we should accept the offer. Plans were made, a moving service was hired, and good-byes were said. We left a lot of family and really good friends behind in Utah. Many of my friends were women I had met in San Francisco or in Salt Lake City when we were all single. We had been blessed to spend a lot of time with each other and had built very strong friendships. Most of us did not have family in Utah and had leaned on each other through the years of single-ness. We had put on each other's wedding showers and baby showers and continued to get together each month for "book club." (I put it in quotes because after a while no one had time to read the book anymore—we just wanted an excuse to catch up and spend time with each other.) I considered these friends to be a family I got to hand-pick before I got married and started my own. I loved them dearly, and they filled my soul every time we got together.

My health had started to get worse and worse around this time. It wasn't bad enough for me to run to a doctor—it was more like a feeling of being "off." I was starting to have problems with brain fog and memory. I always felt like I was stuck in second gear—anxious and revved up. I had gained 40 pounds *after* my daughter was born the year before. I didn't feel like myself mentally. My desire to be social was waning. I just wanted to hunker down and be alone or just with my husband and daughter. The only way to describe this feeling is to imagine yourself rolling up into a protective ball, curling your head down, covering your eyes with your hands and disappearing into a sad darkness.

The move did not help my health. The stress of finding a new home with a toddler in tow, living out of a temporary apartment, having no friends or family nearby, and becoming increasingly incapable of dealing with life took an additional toll on my body. I didn't realize it at the time but I was suffering from many different health issues. I didn't have a doctor in Texas and I just knew all he or she would tell me was that I needed anti-depressants. And looking back to 2004, I was probably right.

My instincts told me there was something wrong that an

anti-depressant wasn't able to fix. My sense of well-being was gone and I felt constantly stressed-out. I didn't want to try to make friends until I knew where we were going to live and what church ward we would be in. What was really happening was that I knew I couldn't be myself and I didn't want anyone to know me that way. I assumed that I would get better and then I could make friends with my normal, happy, functioning self. I was wrong—but could never have known it at the time.

The more stressed and sick I became, the less open and kind I felt. I kept everyone at arm's length to try and protect myself. I was no longer able to trust my judgment on anything. My perceptions of people or situations became more and more muddled. Where I had once had the ability to size up a person and situation rapidly, I could no longer get a 'read' on someone or know if they might be a kindred spirit. My ability to feel connected to God had been declining since 2000. I had no desire to go to church and be among people who could feel things I could no longer relate to. I also lost the memory of who I was, and the ability to talk with others easily. I used to be social, outgoing, energetic, and loved hearing other people's opinions and life stories. As my memory declined and stress increased all I knew was that I wasn't myself. And all I wanted to do was keep everyone out until I could be myself again.

Once we started looking at available homes, we decided we would prefer to build a house and went through the entire planning phase including choosing the lot, exterior, and interior colors and materials. (This is a hugely stressful endeavor by the way—I do not recommend it if you are not well.) My very kind and patient husband and I actually made it through this process only to realize it would take about three months to prep the lot and another five to eight to build the house. This didn't affect my husband too much because he had his office to go to, but for me,

I felt like I was on Pause. The neighborhood we wanted to land in was 20 minutes away from our temporary apartment, and I was not looking forward to driving back and forth with a toddler and spending eight months watching our house sit in various stages of (or lack of) development. Finally, I was so stressed about not being able to feel settled somewhere that we asked the builder if we could transfer our down payment to a recently-built "spec" home. They agreed and we closed on the house and moved in—in 10 days flat. I was so ready to be out of temporary housing and start our new life.

I had hoped that settling somewhere would ease the stress and sickness and I would be able to get well. But it was not to be. If I had had any clue what the next eight years would bring, I would never have made it. It was the most difficult, sad, and depressing existence of loneliness. I became friends with some women in our neighborhood who also had young children. I appreciated their friendship but always knew that the person they thought was me was just a broken shell. I made no friends at church on purpose. I felt I had nothing in common with the women there who could feel a connection to God. We went every Sunday but I felt completely broken down. I did not pray. I did not read my scriptures. There was no rest from the knowledge I was not myself. There was no respite.

Looking back I now realize I was very sick and very depressed. As a result, I isolated myself—which is a classic symptom of depression. The problem was, that after years of sickness and isolation, I was depriving myself of the very thing I needed to get well—OTHER PEOPLE! People with insight, knowledge to share, and a kind ear to listen. People with medical advice or someone who would simply pray for me. People who knew who I was before I became ill and who could help me find my way back. I deprived myself of the very thing I needed most.

In J.K. Rowling's tale of Harry Potter, there is a point where Harry feels like no one understands him. The Ministry of Magic is spreading lies about him to discredit him, and he feels as if no one believes his claims that Voldemort has returned. He is confused, worn-down, and angry. He begins to isolate himself from his friends and wallow in feeling misunderstood. One of my favorite parts of the series is when Luna tells Harry that if she were You-Know-Who, she'd want Harry to feel cut-off from everyone else. She explains that if it's just Harry alone, he is not that much of a threat[48].

The meaning behind that statement speaks volumes. If you were the Adversary, wouldn't you want all of God's children to feel cut-off and alone?

Women are designed to help. We nurture, serve, and care for others. We should band together when things get hard. But what do we do when we begin to suffer? We draw inward and try not to let anyone else see our weakness or pain. When things get really bad inside your head, the last thing you want to do is express your vulnerability. If you can, ask for help. If you can't, keep reading.

From personal dealings with depression and isolation, I know the only way to get out of the round-about is to force some kind of action. It will be hard, but again: you have more power than you realize. Every single time I have pulled out of a depression it was because of ACTION. In the past I have talked with my bishop; I've made changes in my attitude and habits; I forced myself to make new friends; I left a job that was crushing my soul; I changed my diet; I started volunteering at my child's school; I researched good doctors and found one in my area.

I even sought out a good counselor (let's call her Norma) who helped me understand more about these issues. But at one point when it got really bad, I finally had to get on anti-depressants. I *really* did not want to. In fact, Norma and I spent an hour once on the topic of anti-depressants.

I did not want to take them. Period. I knew my body and brain were not in pain because of a need for a pharmaceutical. I needed something else—I just didn't know what it was. I had not made the connection between the gut and the brain at this point. In the meantime, Norma explained to me that after their creation, anti-depressants had allowed thousands of people to leave asylums and lead normal lives and there was no shame in taking them. I explained I had tried once but the prescription made me feel numb. She suggested that particular formula was not a fit for what I needed. Norma also helped me understand that sometimes you have to get your brain in the right place before you can make other changes in your life.

Well, in spite of all my arguments and complete abhorrence at the thought of taking a drug to think and feel better—I did it anyway. And it helped a lot.

Some people need to take them for a few months and then their bodies start working properly again. Others may need to stay on antidepressants for life. I know several of these people, and they are amazingly high-achievers while on their meds—and complete train wrecks off of them. It is absolutely crucial that they have their medication.

There are some things you need to watch out for. The first and biggest mistake people make with antidepressants is when they start taking them, begin feeling great, and then want to get off of them because they are "cured." Do not fall into this trap. You feel cured because the medication is doing what it is supposed to. Follow your doctor's orders and do not wean yourself off of them without supervision.

Antidepressants are powerful, mind-affecting drugs. Do not play Russian roulette with your sanity. Do not get on or off of an antidepressant prescription without working with your doctor. It is a BIG deal. Hopefully after feeling better for a few months you can (together) create a plan to slowly decrease your dosage and see if you tolerate the new dose. If things go well, you could be done with your round of antidepressants and, hopefully, feeling like yourself again. If things don't go well, continue with the prescription and be grateful you don't feel as awful as you did before. You can try decreasing dosages with your doctor's supervision again in the future when you both feel the time is right.

Another thing to watch out for is the antidepressant not working like it should. I have tried five different kinds. Two made me feel numb, one did not work at all, and another made popping effects go off in my brain. None of these symptoms is the desired effect. A fact which seems obvious—except to those who are depressed, can't think straight, and don't know better. However, the last one I tried was golden. I felt much, much better while taking this prescription. In fact, I often wondered to myself, "Is this what *normal* people feel like every day? This is AWESOME!" I felt calm, not overwhelmed, not socially anxious, clear-headed, and like myself. It was wonderful.

I really want to underscore the point that SOMETIMES you need to help your brain so you can focus on fixing the rest of your situation. Your brain drives the body, and if it is not working properly, nothing else will either. There is no shame in getting short (or, in some cases, long-term) boosts of the brain chemicals you need to feel normal. If you keep fighting it like I did, just remember that the Adversary delights in our misery and wants us to feel alone. He knows of the great power for good you could be if you were healthy and well. If you are fighting something that might help you, and you are feeling especially broken and vulnerable, it could be because the Adversary is working especially hard to keep you from getting better.

Just think about it.

Chapter 22
DEPRESSION:
Causes and Cures

Depression affects millions of women every year. It disrupts marriages, childhoods and careers. It also sabotages goals, shatters hopes and crushes dreams. If you or someone you love is mired in its grasp, you are not alone. One out of ten Americans is defined by the Center for Disease Control as depressed. And regardless of whether you deal with mild or overwhelming depression, I send you empathy and compassion. It is truly one of the most difficult afflictions of this mortal existence.

Its causes seem nebulous. Its cures are elusive. But it can be overcome.

Whether depression is the cause of your trials or your problems are the cause of your depression, you may wonder: how do some people stay positive in spite of their troubles? Other people experience great setbacks and seem to escape the grasp of depression. Why is it that some of us cannot seem to find our way out from under the darkness no matter how hard we try? And what do we have to do to overcome depression once and for all? In this chapter we will reveal the answers to these questions.

The Truth Comes Together

There is a reason that the information on how to overcome depression is found at the very end of this book. To truly defeat depression you must first acquaint yourself with the myriad of topics found in earlier chapters. Almost every chapter topic in this book is a cause of depression. And while the origins of depression in today's world are many, the solution comes back to the four pillars of health. You are either malnourished, toxic, overly stressed, or disconnected from others—and for most women, it is a combination of all four. Once you refill your body with nutrients, detoxify both physically and emotionally, dial down the stress, and get connected with others you can win your battle for good.

Unfortunately, the solution is not always simple. Depression is a complex beast and your remedy must be custom tailored to your situation. You are genetically unique, and what will cure someone else may not be the answer for you. Find a good doctor to assist you in your recovery and use the topics in these pages as discussion points. You may also want to find an unbiased third-party to help you gauge your progress.

Below I have included the most likely sources of depression and how to overcome each one. This is your Holy Grail to overcoming depression. Work your way down the list until you feel like yourself again. Do not be afraid of using anti-depressants in the short-term. As stated previously, sometimes you need help to be able to get your head above the water and see the shore. Once you see it, you can stop treading water and start swimming for it. It may seem like a long way away, but you can make it. Trust me—I've been there. Everyone that loves you (myself included) is cheering you on.

And know that nothing feels better than when you reach that sand.

The Depression Top 10: Causes and Cures

1. **Food sensitivities and allergies**; such as gluten intolerance or dairy sensitivity. This is the absolute NUMBER 1 cause of depression because it causes inflammation of the gut lining, malabsorption of vitamins, and inability to manufacture neurotransmitters for the brain. Figure out what your body is fighting against as outlined in the Intolerance and Sensitivity Chapter. Avoid all genetically modified foods. Go on a gut repair diet protocol such as a Paleo plan or Candida-free diet to clean out toxic build up and repair the intestinal lining. This will reset your entire system. Drink one to two high-nutrient smoothies with enzymes each day instead of meals to allow your digestive system to recover. Consume homemade organic bone broths several times a week to heal the gut and provide much-needed minerals. Also take 1 teaspoon of L-glutamine powder in water up to 3 times a day to heal the cilia along your intestinal walls.

2. **Deficiency in B Vitamins.** Specifically B6 and B12 which are found in raw meats and not very shelf-stable—such as inside a vitamin bottle or in a "fortified" packaged food—respectively. B vitamins are crucial for proper brain-chemical formulation and proper cell mitochondria functionality (aka energy). Sublingual forms of B12 are effective for many people, while B shots are helpful to others. Talk with your doctor about these B vitamin injectibles if you have been depressed for long periods of time. They could help jump-start your recovery.

3. **Lack of Vitamin D.** This vitamin/hormone is crucial to proper usage of serotonin within the brain and calcium

levels within the blood. Take a supplement of up to 10,000 IUs a day and lay off the constant use of sunscreen.

4. **Toxicity.** Your body may be backed up with too much junk in its garbage removal system. You could be riddled with heavy metals or candida. Revisit the chapter on Toxicity and follow the guidelines listed there. Quit eating packaged, fried, and preserved food and any undesirable fats (explained in the Fats chapter). Drink a green veggie juice everyday with liver detoxifying additions such as lemons, beets, ginger, and garlic. Take long walks to get your lymph system moving. Fast for 24 hours (and drink lots of water!) a couple of times a month as long as you are not diabetic, pregnant, or nursing. Do a colon cleanse and a liver cleanse as outlined in the chapter on candida. Constipated? Take probiotics and get lots of natural fiber daily. Take extra magnesium if necessary, but get your plumbing working!

5. **Excess stress leading to adrenal fatigue.** Realize that stressing over something is wasted energy. Do what you can to fix things and then leave the rest to God. Analyze and remove some of the things on your "Must Do" list. Take high-quality vitamins, sleep in, get extra Vitamin C, eat good fats and avoid anything fried. Exercise gently and focus on your breathing. Laugh, laugh, and then laugh some more.

6. **Thyroid imbalance.** The thyroid cannot function without iodine, selenium, and other trace minerals. It is also especially burdened by excess gluten consumption and candida toxicity. Get sufficient amounts of trace minerals and omit processed grains and sugar from your diet. Get the following tests done to ensure balanced levels: T3, T4, TSH, Thyroid Antibody Assay, and Reverse T3. Make

sure you have a doctor who understands how to interpret all five tests and why they are important.

7. **Hormones out of balance.** Stress, hormone disrupting toxins, lack of real Vitamin A found in liver meat and cod liver oil, too much sugar, and a lack of essential vitamins and minerals throw your hormones off. You must reduce stress so the adrenals quit stealing your pregnenalone to make cortisol instead of other necessary hormones. De-stress, eat good fats (especially Omega-3's, cod liver oil, and borage oil) and eat good food. Take a high-quality multi-vitamin supplement for all the micro nutrients we are missing in our soils that aren't making it into our food supply. Detoxify your make-up bag and medicine cabinet to remove phthalates and parabens. Consume extra cruciferous veggies to clean out your estrogen receptors. Sleep.

8. **Insomnia.** Not sleeping properly affects every aspect of your life. Things seem overwhelming when they normally wouldn't be. Exercise in the morning. Do yoga. Avoid caffeine at all costs. Make sure you are getting plenty of Vitamin D as mentioned above. Take 400 mg magnesium and/or 2-5 gms of melatonin 30 minutes before bed. Pure, high-quality lavender essential oil placed on the bottoms of your feet at night is also very helpful. You may need some bio-identical hormones to get your sleep cycles working again. If you are taking pure T4 for thyroid issues, you may need some natural T3 to lower your reverse T3 (RT3) in order to allow your hormones, adrenals, and cycles to rebalance and dreams to return.

9. **Unresolved emotional issues and negative thoughts.** Everyone has emotional issues, but yours may be exceptionally heavy to bear. Abuse and neglect affect your thought patterns and self-esteem in many ways. Find a

good counselor. Learn how to do "The Work" by Byron Katie as explained in the Compromised Thoughts and Mental Maintenance chapter. Get repatterned as explained in the Resonance Repatterning chapter. You can't fix problems that you don't know exist. Heal the past hurts, and know the future doesn't have to reflect the past.

10. **Loneliness and isolation.** To make a friend you need to show up. Go to every work, church, and/or school activity you possibly can. Volunteer. Ask someone to lunch. If they are "busy" more than twice, ask somebody else. If you can't summon the courage or energy to do any of these things, specifically pray for new friends to come into your life and ask others who love you to do the same. There are plenty of lonely people on this planet—solve your issue and theirs at the same time!

11. **A Bonus Topic: Dehydration.** You may not even realize how desperately your body needs more water. Diet sodas, caffeine, excessive sodium, preservatives, unhealthy fats, and other toxins all affect the delicate fluid balance within our cells. Omitting the above will allow the water you drink to get to the places it needs to go. One doctor I visited listed the top 3 problems of all her patients to be: 1) Food intolerances, 2) Lack of sleep, and 3) DEHYDRATION. So avoid the no-no list above, get hydrated, and stay that way.

At the Close

For the record, I personally grappled with every single problem on the list above. I know what it feels like to want to leave this world. Any one of the above items by themselves can leave you in a state of despair, but when you combine any number of them, life can seem no longer worth living. However, from personal experience, I know they can all be overcome. It is my hope that with the above list, you will find your way back to health as fast as possible. And know that God's assistance will always be given to those who struggle. *Never* give up!

In the Harry Potter series, J.K. Rowling writes of "dementors" who extract the happiness out of people. The characters in the book say that when dementors attack, the victims feel as if they will "never be cheerful again." After an assault, chocolate helps the afflicted to recover. Does any of that sound familiar? In an interview, Ms. Rowling admitted the dementors were created from her personal bouts with depression. She struggled as she wrote the first book in a small apartment with a new baby, all on her own, while living on government assistance. But with time and healing, she pushed forward to raise a family and author one of the greatest series ever written. Think of what would have been lost if she had abandoned hope.

If you are overwhelmed, ask for help. Your church advisors, family doctor, or a professional counselor are all good places to start. Depression is not your fault, and you do not have to bear this burden by yourself. **You matter. Your life matters. Your challenges matter.** And I send you support and encouragement.

The Adversary is attacking women mercilessly. From our altered food supply, to broken communities and feelings of isolation, to being constantly stressed, we have serious threats to our happiness, health, and fertility. But we also have limitless power at our command. We now know the enemy's tactics and game plan. It is time for us to rise up and fight back. Change what you eat. Vote with every food dollar you spend. Detoxify your body and your life. Lend a hand to those who suffer. Be kind to yourself and others and realize that every person struggles with something you know nothing about.

With the information you hold in your hand (or on your screen), you now have the power to:

Heal your body.

Heal your mind.

Reconnect with God.

And change the world for the better—one person at a time.

Chapter 23
KNOWLEDGE IS RELATIVE

Throughout my health journey, I read a lot of books. Books on health, books on nutrition, books on good fortune, books on business matters, books on attitude and mental fortitude, books on financial markets and statistical analysis (I have done financial planning and analysis by profession), and books on God and Christ. I absorbed a lot of information—a lot. And as my mind and body healed, I was actually able to remember some of it.

I was also blessed with access to one of the most brilliant men I have ever met, who just happens to be my husband. He is confident without arrogance, patient beyond belief, and funny to boot. He is also an amazing problem-solver. I learned more from our conversations and philosophizing than from any university class I have ever taken.

What I realized after reading all these books and other sources of data is this: intelligence is innate. That's right, it's inside of you. We may chase after advanced degrees—and we should certainly strive to educate ourselves and become knowledgeable people—but at the end of the day, if you have access to God, you have the best learning resource available. His Spirit will testify to you of correct principles as you learn, whether they are temporal or spiritual. It will warn you of upcoming danger. If you are on the right spiritual channel, you can discern good ideas from bad ones and act accordingly. God will not always tell you what to do, but that's where you get to stretch and grow and decide for yourself. It is not easy in today's hectic world, but slowing down to listen to Him is the smartest thing we can ever do.

Do know that this seemingly negative attitude towards higher learning comes from a type-A, finals-driven student who did graduate from college. I do not disrespect learning done in universities. But too many people today are wrapped up in the misconception that university learning is the only path to success. Many place their belief in a degree instead of God. His Spirit could guide you to pursue a trade or other means of supporting yourself and your family. In today's world, tradesmen and women often make higher incomes than college graduates drowning in debt. If anything ever happens to crash our current society, those with a trade will be better equipped to forge ahead in a new world. Either way, learning is a lifelong process no matter what the venue, and we should never stop striving to educate ourselves, regardless of whether we have a college diploma or not.

My education taught me a lot and opened doors of employment, to be sure—but it also taught me that a degree doesn't determine your self-worth. Neither does having straight A's, a perfect body weight, or being the most amazing athlete or musician on the planet. Without the Spirit to underline which of that you've learned is actually true and important, no talent or hard-earned goal is valued in the proper perspective. In fact, for many of the past ten years, due to my poor health I was unable to remember hardly anything I had learned in years past. To say it was humiliating to go from feeling somewhat smart to barely being able to remember my children's names would be an understatement. But from this humiliation I learned that self-worth is not determined by how much we know, but by how much we strive to press forward, draw closer to Christ, and love others.

Recently I read a book on mathematical modeling and how accurately (or inaccurately) these models actually predict events. It was a long, rather tedious, read. The gist of the book was this: that all the geniuses in the world cannot accurately predict the stock market, geological calamities, or acts of war—even if they think they can. I enjoyed the book because it underscored what I had begun to believe in college: that *all* economists and analysts run predictive equations based on some kind of assumption—and assumptions are almost always wrong. When the underlying assumption that the research is based on is incorrect, the foundation is broken and the results built on that foundation are skewed at best. In the end, the most educated predictions are just a gamble. It's all Vegas, baby. In my opinion the most enlightening thing the author said was simply, "be prepared for anything." Now that IS good advice—and I bet he didn't need multiple advanced degrees to figure that out.

But in spite of the fact that the author was blowing the whistle on predictive modeling and those that thought they were smarter than God, what I couldn't help feeling as I read this book was an annoyance at the author's analytical pontifications. It was too much mind and far too little spirit. If you drew 3 circles with the labels: Mind, Body, and Spirit that intersect in the middle; his mind circle was far too large. It pushed aside the other two circles and put him out of balance and far from the source of his innate intelligence—his spirit. I finally realized that the reason I was so annoyed by this imbalance was because I had done the exact same thing for years while trying to regain my health. (If something really bothers you about someone else, it is often an indicator that you are looking at one of your own shortcomings.)

I began my journey with a laser-focused determination to

discover what breaks down the female body and to heal myself, and many helpful and worthwhile things were certainly learned. But by the end, I realized it was my spirit that was out of balance. I had harbored resentments and separated myself from God because of the pain I had experienced seemingly without assistance. As a result of holding on to my resentment, I endured my trials with a bitter heart and a body that could not heal.

The assumptions I based my results on were wrong. God never leaves any of His children without assistance. Sometimes it just appears that way because we have to learn from our trials. God gave me a supportive husband and loving family to aid me in my struggles. I also had old friends re-enter my life right when I needed them to help me get through especially difficult times. I chose to see things from a bleak perspective because my mind wanted to be in control. In my pain, I chose to dive into facts and figures to try and heal. From my chase of temporal knowledge, I began to truly understand the scripture 2 Nephi 9:28 in the Book of Mormon: "When they are learned they think they are wise, and they hearken not unto the counsel of God, for they set it aside, supposing they know of themselves, wherefore, their wisdom is foolishness and it profiteth them not."

My mother has always wanted a college degree. She thinks that to be truly smart you need a degree. All three of her children graduated from college, and she is very proud of her kids. But what I want her, and every man and woman like her, to know is this: You have everything you need already inside of you—just like the Scarecrow in the Wizard of Oz. If you want to learn something, read books about it or take a class. Then share what you've learned with others. It is the best way to retain information. If you want to start a business, learn from other business owners. Network—people are your best source of information (and most love to share). Even better, you won't end up tens of thousands of dollars in debt from school loans, and you may make some life-long friends in the process. And never let the Adversary or anyone else make you think less of yourself. You are already amazing—you were born that way.

For the record, my mother is the kindest, most God-loving, and full-of-wonder person you could ever hope to meet. I think when it comes to loving others and having great faith, she is far superior to any college graduate I know. Somehow, I think God values this far more highly than any degree. In many near-death experiences I have studied, the authors describe being able to learn and comprehend vast amounts of book data instantaneously after death—but faith and experience is earned. That's why we are here!

The point of all this is to help you to heal by removing the stress of talking down to yourself. Spiritually, we all depend on Heavenly Father, regardless of how accomplished or great we think we are. The problem among women is that we don't think we are great. We often get stuck in a negative-thinking downward spiral that leads to depression and lack of action or worse: frantic energy spent running in the wrong direction. The example I used above was academic, but the same thing applies to accomplished business men and women, musicians, actors, lawyers, and politicians.

It's hard to be a rock star and not think you are God's Gift to the Planet. This over-confidence most surely puts the mind part of the equation out of balance with the body and spirit. But on the flip side, as women we sometimes feel that if we are not rock star mothers or PTA presidents or extremely accomplished in one of the above-listed professions, we are nothing. And nothing could be farther from the truth.

If you feel like one of the "un-talented," I can promise you that you do not see yourself clearly. This may sound like boring rhetoric, but I must remind you of a universal truth: You are a divine child of God and were born to do something no one else can do. You may not realize what it is yet, but it is there and is part of your life plan. Every trial you have adds to your ability to accomplish it. Cherish the unfolding of your plan and know that all is well. You don't need to be anything other than the light that you are. Gently and persistently strive for the best things, to be sure—but first, make sure you refocus on what those best things are. "Ask, and it shall be given you. Seek and ye shall find; knock and it shall be opened unto you" (Mathew 7:7).

I wish you all the best in your quest for health. May your journey be short and your life be filled with joy.

With love,
Wanda Cooper

EPILOGUE

I always get distracted during movies when the guy asks the girl out for a date and they never name a time or a place. I always wonder: How do they know when and where to meet? *Details*, people!

Along the same lines, I do not want to leave you hanging on the specific details of how I was actually healed, just in case you wanted to know.

All of the chapters in this book were discovered through layers of personal suffering. I really only started healing when I began a nutritional supplementation regimen, altered my diet to avoid food sensitivities, and stuck with it. I also had to get my thyroid medications balanced. It turns out that my body doesn't convert T4 to T3 well and as a result, it created a lot of Reverse T3 that clogged my cell receptors. Adding T3 to my daily regimen (also known as Liothyronine or Cytomel) lowered my reverse T3 levels and along with it went my insomnia and social anxiety. I also take bio-identical progesterone during the latter half of my monthly cycle to assist with sleep and avoiding PMS.

The depression lifted to a large degree after I removed wheat from my diet for three months. It was only then that I was able to feel joy again. I needed a lot of healing and nutrients to overcome the abuse I had inflicted upon my intestines. (Recall that I was told five years earlier that I was intolerant to gluten. I just couldn't muster the mental strength to avoid it at that time.) I have never been officially diagnosed with Celiac disease but would not be surprised if I have it.

For the record, I took a lot of wrong turns to figure out what really worked. Being stubborn is good in some ways and terrible in others. Because it took me so long to discover and apply the methods held in this book, I endured decades of damage to my body. To be completely honest, I feel very fortunate to be alive. The fact I am still around to raise my children is a blessing and I give thanks for it every day. And while I feel worlds better than I used to, my health still has its minor ups and downs.

My previous battle with cancer, genetic weakness at clearing toxins, and prolonged experiences with stress and malnutrition mean that cancer could rear its ugly head again. If that happens, or some other health issue affects my life, I want you to know it is not because the protocols in this book don't work. It will be because I unknowingly (and sometimes, knowingly) damaged my body through stress and neglect for over 40 years before I turned things around.

But for now, I truly feel joy, energy, and a passion for living. And it is my goal in life to help others feel the same.

The nutritional supplements I take have to support all the weak points in my genetic structure and the former abuses I inflicted on my body: adrenal burn-out, poor detoxification pathways, absence of a thyroid because of cancer, and severe malnutrition from damaged intestinal walls. I take the following nutritional supplements daily:

- Usana Essentials Multivitamin (2 chelated minerals and 2 antioxidant caps twice a day)
- Nordic Naturals ProOmega fish oil (1 cap)
- Priority One Adrenoplex (1-2 caps a day) to help rebuild and support my adrenals

- NuMedica C-Bioflav 1000 (1 cap) to further support the adrenals
- Vitamin D3 cholicalciferol 1000 IU
- Green Pastures Blue Ice Royal Butter Oil/Fermented Cod Liver Oil Blend (3-9 caps)
- Magnesium chelate (600 mg)
- Coral calcium (800 mg)

I drink a scoop of VegeSplash apple-carrot flavor with a tbsp. of powdered L-glutamine in 8 ounces of water each morning to detoxify excess estrogens. I also take enzymes with every meal and a super high count probiotic (225 billion) every other day.

My health situation is extreme. I only feel good when I exercise often, avoid wheat, sugar, bad fats, and genetically modified foods covered in pesticides, and take all my supplements. I hope that your situation will not get as bad as mine. I pray that you will use the information in this book to avoid damaging your body past a point of no return.

I did every cleanse and detox protocol mentioned in this book and found them all to be helpful in their own right. But the one cleanse that made the largest difference was the candida protocol. It was extremely hard to stick to, but had the greatest effect on clearing my mind, skin, and balancing my hormones. I have decided that for me, sugar is problematic and try to avoid it whenever possible.

I still hate cooking. As a mom, I have to force myself to accommodate everyone's preferences and individual food intolerances. And I do so, because I love my family. In our house, we try to eat very healthy meals at home and we splurge (to a degree) when we travel or eat out. It is next to impossible to control the types of fats you eat at restaurants, so I try to minimize eating at fried food places and restaurants that use low-quality ingredients whenever possible. But from learning the hard way, I do not eat wheat—no matter what.

I was also blessed to finally be able to make some new friends in my community. As I healed, I was able to feel like myself again and create connections with others. Having more social outlets was a huge boon to my recovery and it fed positively upon itself to create additional opportunities to connect with even more people.

But without the consistency of love and support from my husband, none of this progress would have been possible. He picked up the pieces with the kids when I could not function. He made me laugh when I no longer thought it was possible. And he financially supported all the doctor visits and medical expenses and never complained. He is my best friend and deserves far more credit than I can capture on this page. He is the steady, reassuring voice of reason in our home and I am lovingly grateful for him—always.

I began to rebuild my relationship with God slowly as my body healed. It did not happen overnight. When you experience misery beyond what you thought possible, it takes time to restore your faith in God and belief that there are good things in this world. With time and prayer, I began to feel that perhaps there was a reason for all the suffering. That belief led me to write this book. And one day, I hope to glimpse the bigger picture of God's intention.

The most important thing I learned from this experience is to *keep trying*—even if all you can do is drag one foot around the other. Because eventually, the rain stops and the clouds pass. And when the sun finally reappears, it brings more joy and gratitude than before. And my favorite thing in life these days?

Without a doubt—it's the rainbows.

There is a lot more information that
I wanted to share with you, but at some point
I have to stop writing so you can actually
read the book. So instead, I created a
website and blog to capture the rest.

For helpful lists on fats, supplements, and
other tips and stories, please visit my website at

www.brokenvesselrestored.com

REFERENCES

1   Job 38: 7, Old Testament, The Bible

2   Moses 4:2, Pearl of Great Price

3   Moses 4:3-4, Pearl of Great Price

4   Genesis 3:15, Old Testament, The Bible

5   1 Corinthinans 2:14, The Bible, New Testament; Mosiah 3:19, The Book of Mormon; Moses 6:49, The Pearl of Great Price

6   Sally Fallon. *Nourishing Traditions*. New Trends Publishing, Washington DC, 2001. Pg. xv

7   Julie Cart, "Study Finds Utah Leads Nation in Antidepressant Use," *Los Angeles Times,* 20 February 2002, A6.

8   Junger, Alejandro, M.D. Clean Gut. New York: HarperOne Harper Collins Publishers, 2013. Pg 43.

9   Tolmunen, T. et al. 2007. Dietary folate and depressive symptoms are associated in middle-aged Finnish men. *J. Nutr* 133 (10):3233-3236.

10 Penninx, B. W., et al. 2000. Vitamin B(12) deficiency and depression in physically disabled older women: Epidemiologic evidence from the Women's Health and Aging Study. *Am J Psychiatry* 157 (5):715-21.

11 Roundup® is a registered trademark of Monsanto Company

12 Smith, Jeffrey M. Genetic Roulette. Fairfield, IA. Yes! Books, 2007.

13 Singh, Man Mohan. "Wheat Gluten as a Pathogenic Factor in Schizophrenia." *Science* 191.4225 (1976): 401-402.

14 William Davis, M.D. *Wheat Belly.* Rodale, New York. 2011. Pg 53.

15 Fontana, Luigi, et al. "Visceral Fat Adipokine Secretion is Associated with Systemic Inflammation in Obese Humans." *Diabetes* 56.4 (2007): 1010-1013.

16 Kuk, Jennifer L., et al. "Visceral Fat Is an Independent Predictor of All-cause Mortality in Men." *Obesity* 14.2 (2006): 336-341.

17 Jenkins, D. J., et al. "Glycemic Index of Foods: a Physiological Basis

for Carbohydrate Exchange." *The American Journal of Clinical Nutrition* 34.3 (1981): 362-366.

18 Nelsen Jr, David A. "Gluten-sensitive Enteropathy (celiac disease): More Common Than You Think." *American Family Physician* 66.12 (2002): 2259-2266.

19 According to the work of Dr. Alessio Fasano, M.D. Medical Director for the Center for Celiac Research

20 Roundup® is a registered trademark of Monsanto Company

21 Samsel and Seneff. Journal of Interdisciplinary Toxicology (Vol. 6(4): 159-184).

22 Itan Yuval, PhD, et al., "A Worldwide Correlation of Lactase Persistence Phenotype and Genotypes", *BMC Evolutionary Biology*, Feb. 9, 2010

23 Food and Drug Administration "BST Update: First Year Experience Reports," Mar. 14, 1995

24 Smith, Jeffrey M. Genetic Roulette. Fairfield, IA. Yes! Books, 2007.

25 MLA Adebamowo, Clement A., et al. "Milk Consumption and Acne in Adolescent Girls." (2006).

26 MLA Biro, Frank M., et al. "Pubertal Assessment Method and Baseline Characteristics in a Mixed Longitudinal Study of Girls." *Pediatrics* 126.3 (2010): e583-e590.

27 MLA Panush, Richard S., Robert M. Stroud, and Ella M. Webster. "Food-Induced (allergic) Arthritis. Inflammatory Arthritis Exacerbated by Milk." *Arthritis & Rheumatism* 29.2 (1986): 220-226.

28 Oomen, Claudia M., et al. "Association between trans fatty acid intake and 10-year risk of coronary heart disease in the Zutphen Elderly Study: a prospective population-based study." *The Lancet* 357.9258 (2001): 746-751.

29 Mozaffarian, Dariush, et al. "Dietary intake of trans fatty acids and systemic inflammation in women." *The American journal of clinical nutrition* 79.4 (2004): 606-612.

30 Salmeron, Jorge, et al. "Dietary fat intake and risk of type 2 diabetes in women." *The American journal of clinical nutrition* 73.6 (2001): 1019-1026.

31 Portillo, María P., et al. "Modifications induced by dietary lipid source in adipose tissue phospholipid fatty acids and their consequences in lipid mobilization." *British Journal of Nutrition* 82.04 (1999): 319-327. Dulloo, Abdul G., et al. "Differential effects of high-fat diets varying in fatty acid composition on the efficiency of lean and fat tissue deposition during weight recovery after low food intake." *Metabolism* 44.2 (1995): 273-279.

32 Kabara, J. J. "The Pharmacological Effects of Lipids, The American Oil Chemists Society, Champaign, IL, 1978, 1-14; Cohen, LA, et al." *J Natl Cancer Inst* 77 (1986): 43.

33 T. Colin Campbell and Thomas M. Campbell II, The China Study. (Dallas: Benbella Books, Inc.) 21, 255-268.

34 T. Colin Campbell and Thomas M. Campbell II, The China Study. (Dallas: Benbella Books, Inc.) 291, 397.

35 Eritsland, Jan. "Safety considerations of polyunsaturated fatty acids." *The American journal of clinical nutrition* 71.1 (2000): 197S-201S. "Process of stabilizing fatty materials containing oleic acid and higher polyunsaturated fatty acids." U.S. Patent 2,435,159, issued January 27, 1948.

36 Beasley, Joseph D., and Jerry Swift. "The Kellogg report: the impact of nutrition, environment and lifestyle on the health of Americans." (1989).

37 Felton, C. V., et al. "Dietary polyunsaturated fatty acids and composition of human aortic plaques." *The Lancet* 344.8931 (1994): 1195-1196.

38 H. Petousis-Harris, "Saturated Fat Has Been Unfairly Demonised: Yes," *Primary Health Care* 3, no. 4 (December 1, 2011): 317-319.

39 See the work of George Macilwain, *The General Nature and Treatment of Tumors*. London, UK. John Churchill, 1845. Also see the work of Dr. Max Gershon, *A Cancer Therapy: The Results of 50 Cases*, 1958.

40 Am J Clin Nutr **December 2003** vol. 78 no. 6 **1128-1134**

41 Mühlbauer B, Schwenk M, Coram WM, Antonin KH, Etienne P, Bieck PR, Douglas FL. Magnesium-L-aspartate-HCl and magnesium-oxide: bioavailability in healthy volunteers. Eur J Clin Pharmacol 1991;40:437-8.

Lindberg JS, Zobitz MM, Poindexter JR, Pak CY. Magnesium bioavailability from magnesium citrate and magnesium oxide. J Am Coll Nutr 1990;9:48-55.

Walker AF, Marakis G, Christie S, Byng M. Mg citrate found more bioavailable than other Mg preparations in a randomized, double-blind study. Mag Res 2003;16:183-91.

42 Sally Fallon. *Nourishing Traditions*. New Trends Publishing, Washington DC, 2001. Pg. 16.

43 Klein S, et al. Progressive Alterations in lipid and glucose metabolism during short-term fasting in young adult men. American Journal of Physiology 1993; 265 (Endocrinology and metabolism 28):E801-E806

44 Krumholz, Harlan M., et al. "Lack of association between cholesterol and coronary heart disease mortality and morbidity and all-cause mortality in persons older than 70 years." *JAMA: The Journal of the American Medical Association* 272.17 (1994): 1335-1340.

45 de Lau, Lonneke ML, et al. "Serum cholesterol levels and the risk of Parkinson's disease." *American Journal of Epidemiology* 164.10 (2006): 998-1002.

46 West, Rebecca, et al. "Better memory functioning associated with higher total and LDL cholesterol levels in very elderly subjects without the APOE4 allele." *The American Journal of Geriatric Psychiatry: Official Journal of the American Association for Geriatric Psychiatry* 16.9 (2008): 781.

47 Brené Brown. *Daring Greatly*. Penguin Group Inc. New York, 2012. Pg 145.

48 I scoured *Harry Potter and The Order of the Phoenix* to try and find the exact words J.K. Rowling used, but alas, it turns out these lines were spoken by Luna in the fifth *movie* of the series. They came from the screenwriters who adapted the book to film. Regardless of origin, the words Luna's character delivered hit me like a ton of bricks.

INDEX

C

L

M

R

S

T

CPSIA information can be obtained at www.ICGtesting.com
Printed in the USA
LVOW01s0620170714

394646LV00001B/1/P